AF564555

AVIAN PATHOLOGY

NIPA® GENX ELECTRONIC RESOURCES & SOLUTIONS P. LTD.
New Delhi-110 034

About the Authors

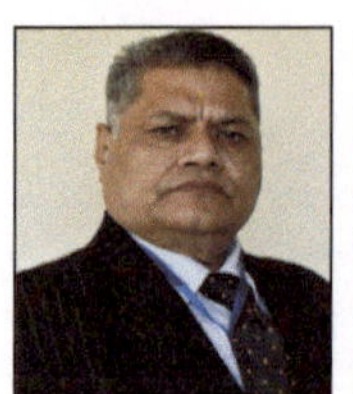

Prof RS Chauhan – Cowpathy Man, MVSc, PhD, FNAVS FSIIP, FIAVP, Diplomat ICVP, PDCR, ACPPM, OCTT MBA EX-Director ICAR-IVRI, JD CADRAD, Director IBT National Fellow, Advisor WHO. Member, Animal Welfare Board of India; Member, CPCSEA (Govt. of India); Chairman Scientific Advisory Committee, ICMR-NARFBR.

Born on September 10th, 1958 in a farmer's family, Dr. Chauhan completed his Bachelors (80.3%) with honours, Master (85.8%) and Doctoral degree (90.0%) in Veterinary Sciences with specialization in veterinary pathology from G.B. Pant University of Agric. & Tech., Pantnagar. He served the country in various capacities including Assistant Professor/ADIO (1983-96), Associate Professor (1996-1999), National Fellow (1999-2004) and Joint Director (CADRAD), IVRI, Izatnagar(2004-2009), Director & Vice-Chancellor(2009), ICAR-IVRI and Campus Director, IBT, Patwadangar (2009-2013). During his tenure as academician and scientist, he has written 112 books including 35 manuals and 1 monograph very popular among the students world over. He contributed 99 chapters in different books and published 235 research and 59 review papers. Besides, he participated in International / National Conferences and presented 178 papers. He is life member of 15 scientific bodies and has been in several executive committee such as Chairman, Panch Gavya Professionals' Club; President, Cow Therapy Society; Secretary-General, Society for Immunology and Immunopathology; Vice President, Indian Society of Veterinary Educators; Zonal Secretary, Indian Association of Veterinary Pathologists and Joint Secretary, Indian Virology Society, President, Dr. J.L. Vegad Foundation, Expert Member Research Group, Committee for Certification of Pathologists, Vice-President, IAVP; Registrar, ICVP, etc.

Based on his contributions and scientific achievements, he has been awarded with several prizes, medals and honours including Best Young Scientist Award (1992), IAAVR Award (1996), National Fellow Award (1999), Fellow NAVS (2000), Fellow SIIP (2001), K.S. Nair Memorial Award (1999), Vigyan Bharti Award (2000), Dr. C.M. Singh Trust Award (2002), Dr. Rajendra Prasad Award (2002), Shri Ramlal Agrawal National Award (2000), Best Paper Award SIIP (2003), Best Paper Award IAVA (2001, 2002, 2003), Best Teacher Award (2004) by GBPUAT, Fellow, IAVP (2006), Gopal Gaurav (2007), Bharat Excellence Award (2007), Diplomat, ICVP (2008), Intas-ISVE Best Veterinary Scientist Award (2008), Best Academician Award (2012), Moropant Pingle Go Sewa National Award (2015), Outstanding Scientist Award (2019), Research Excellence Award (2020), Indo Asian-Claude Bourgelat Distinguished Innovative Scientist Award-2020 in Animal Immunopathology and MAN OF COWPATHY at GADVASU Ludhiana etc. in recognition of his research and teaching endeavor. He has been inducted in many national and international scientific/advisory committees and boards including Member, WHO/IPCS Committee on Environmental Health Criteria. Dr. Chauhan added many new including Enterotoxaemia, Pyometra, ETEC infection in camels, isolated camel pox virus, developed rapid diagnostic test DIA for the first time in India. He reported role of cell mediated immunity in rotavirus infection in calves. His pioneer work includes immunopathology due to pesticides, heavy metals, mycotoxins and nanoparticles. Dr. Chauhan developed a new method using MTT dye for detection of CMI response. He has scientifically validated Panchgavya and named it as "Cowpathy".

He have been recognized internationally as visiting Professor, University of Wageningen and Advisor, WHO. Dr. Chauhan guided more than 50 scholars for their Masters and Doctoral research; most of them are placed as Professors, Scientists, Officers in Indian Army, banks and industry in India and abroad. At present he is working as Head Veterinary Pathology, Chairman Scientific Advisory Committee ICMR-NARFBR, Member AWBI and CPCSEA (Govt of India). Prof Chauhan superannuated on 30th June 2024 after distinguish service of 41.5 years and still contributing to the profession through lectures, writings and research and particularly developing literature/ books for the benefit of students and young generation.

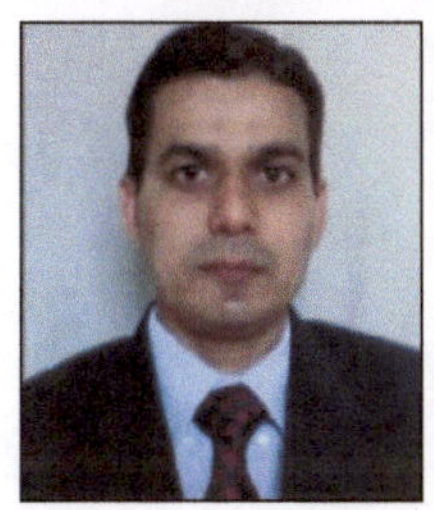

(Dr.) Desh Deepak Singh is Veterinary Graduate and Post Graduate in Veterinary Pathology from College of Veterinary and Animal Sciences, Govind Ballabh Pant University of Agriculture and Technology (GBPUA&T), Pantnagar (Uttarakhand) India in 2001 and 2003. He was awarded outstanding PG student award by GBPUA&T, Pantnagar in 2003. He visited Istanbul, Turkey to present research paper in world poultry congress-2004. He joined as Assistant Professor, Department of Veterinary Pathology, College of Veterinary Sciences & Animal Husbandry, Acharya Narendra Dev University of Agriculture & Technology (ANDUA&T), Kumarganj, Ayodhya, Uttar Pradesh in 2004. He completed his Ph.D. as in-service candidate from U. P. Pandit Deen Dayal Upadhyaya Pashu Chikitsa Vigyan Vishwavidyalaya Evam Go Anusandhan Sansthan (DUVASU), Mathura, Uttar Pradesh, India and promoted to Associate Professor in ANDUA&T, Kumarganj, Ayodhya. Prof. Singh was selected as Professor, Veterinary Pathology, DUVASU, Mathura and presently working as Professor & Head, Department of Veterinary Pathology, UP Veterinary University (DUVASU), Mathura, Uttar Pradesh. He is having more than 20 years' experience of teaching Undergraduate (UG) and Postgraduate (PG) courses of Veterinary Pathology along with vast experience of disease diagnosis, research and extension. He has published more than 55 original research papers in referred journals, 04 books, 04 laboratory manuals for Under Graduate students, 02 manuals for Veterinary Officers, 08 review articles, 10 book chapters and 54 technical/popular articles. He was awarded young scientist award by Society of Immunology and Immunopathology; Prakash best poster award; best poster award by Indian Association of

Veterinary Pathology (IAVP); best paper presentation award by Indian Society of Veterinary Anatomy; best poster award by UP chapter of Indian Society of Veterinary Surgery; best paper award in National Conference held at ANDUA&T, Kumarganj, Ayodhya, Uttar Pradesh; Best poster and best oral presentation award by Indian Society of Veterinary Pharmacology and Toxicology (ISVPT). Prof. Singh is life member of Indian Association of Veterinary Pathologists (IAVP) since 2002; Society of Immunology and Immunopathology (SIIP), Indian Association of Veterinary Public Health Specialists (IAVPHS).

AVIAN PATHOLOGY

R.S. Chauhan
M.V.Sc., Ph.D. (Path.), FNAVS, FSIIP, FIAVP, PDCR, OCTT, ACPPM, MBA
(Ex- Advisor WHO, Ex- Director IVRI, Ex-JDCADRAD, Ex-Director IBT
Ex- National Fellow ICAR)
Member Animal Welfare Board of India (Govt. of India)
Member, CCSEA (Govt of India)
Chairman, SAC, NARFBR (ICMR)
Ex-Professor and Head, Department of Veterinary Pathology
GB Pant University of Agriculture & Technology Pantnagar - 263 145
Uttarakhand, India

Desh Deepak Singh
M.V.Sc., Ph.D.
Professor and Head
Department of Veterinary Pathology
U. P. Pandit Deen Dayal Upadhyaya Pashu Chikitsa Vigyan Vishwavidyalaya Evam
Go Anusandhan, Sansthan (DUVASU), Mathura-281001, Uttar Pradesh, India

NIPA® GENX ELECTRONIC RESOURCES & SOLUTIONS P. LTD.
New Delhi-110 034

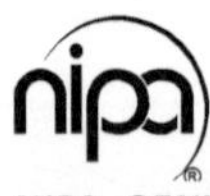

NIPA® GENX ELECTRONIC
RESOURCES & SOLUTIONS P. LTD.
101,103, Vikas Surya Plaza, CU Block
L.S.C.Market, Pitam Pura, New Delhi-110 034
Ph : +91 11 4386 0225, 9717133558, 9540816132
E-mail: newindiapublishingagency@gmail.com
Website: www.niparesources.com

Print ISBN 978-93-58874-25-9

ebook ISBN: 978-93-58875-62-1

Composed and Designed by NIPA®.

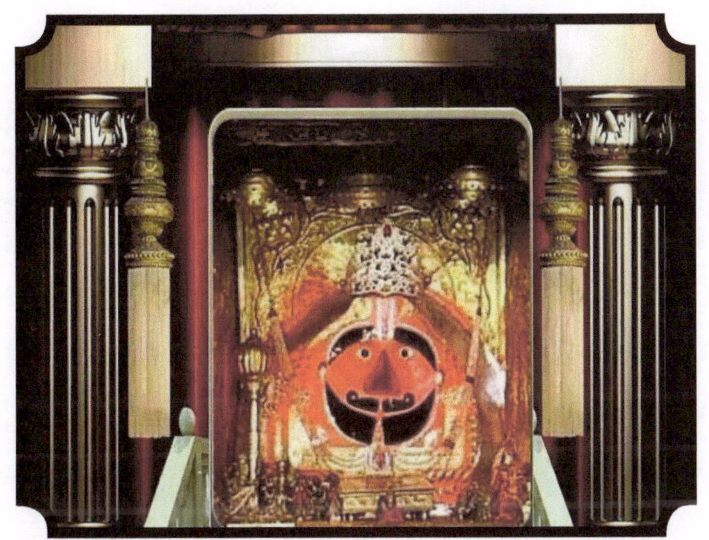

**Dedicated to Anjani Nandan
Pavansut Lord Hanuman**

Preface

Veterinary Pathology is an important discipline of Veterinary Sciences which makes a bridge in between the basic and clinical sciences. The knowledge of Veterinary Pathology makes the Veterinarian a perfect diagnostician particularly when his patients (animal and birds) can't speak their illness to the doctor. Keeping in view the need of study of Veterinary Pathology to become a good Veterinary doctor, the book "Avian Pathology" is written for the use of teachers, students and field veterinarians. The complexity of the subject is presented in a simplified way particularly keeping the view of Indian geo-climatic conditions and poultry population. However, students of Veterinary Science desire a compact text of Avian Pathology covering the VCI new syllabus of pathology which can be utilized during their study and examinations particularly in competitive examinations. Hence, this textbook is prepared as a text material to all those who want to know Avian Pathology at undergraduate and postgraduate level and are interested in any kind of competitive examination or interview. It covers all the topics of pathology of avian diseases. The text is described in a very simple format including avian inflammation; nutritional disorders; pathology of bacterial; viral; fungal; parasitic chlamydial; spirochaetal; mycoplasmal diseases along with vices and miscellaneous disease conditions with their etiology, clinical manifestations, characteristic macroscopic and microscopic features along with diagnosis; only salient features are mentioned avoiding detailed text. Hope this book "Avian Pathology" not only will find a place in the young fraternity of Veterinary Science but also it will be highly useful to the field Veterinarians for diagnosing diseases on the basis of characteristic clinical manifestations, and lesions and in writing of post mortem report of poultry. The help rendered by our colleagues and students in preparation and designing of this book is duly acknowledged. Readers' comments are welcome to further improve the book.

Authors

Contents

1

Avian Inflammation

• Avian Inflammation

Inflammation is a process which begins following a sublethal injury to tissue and ends with complete healing or death. It is characterized by five cardinal signs. Cardinal signs of inflammation are:

- Redness
- Heat
- Swelling
- Pain
- Loss of function
- Inflammation is beneficial in most of cases expect
- In prolonged or unending process
- In inflammation of immunological origin i.e. hypersensitivity and autoimmunity.
- It provides basic foundation of pathogenesis and pathology.
- It is now said that immunity is the resistance of body, while inflammation is the process by which the immune mechanism are implemented.
- The basis of inflammation remains same be it mammal or birds. For details, one can refer the chapter inflammation and heading in book "Illustrated Veterinary Pathology". However, there are some differences in reaction in birds which are briefly listed below:

1. Adult bird has greater capacity to react in comparison to embryos and chicks
2. In birds, there is increased permeability in venules. While in mammals it occurs in capillary/ arterioles.

3. In poultry, Heterophils are the first line of defence and comes first in inflammation followed by mononuclear cells. However, in mammals the sequence is not clear.
4. In poultry, Basophils are seen in significant numbers at the site in early stage of inflammation. These cells degranulate to release histamine. However, in mammals basophils are rarely seen.
5. Formation of perivascular foci due to infiltration of lymphoid cells causing cuffing around blood vessels. This is very common in avian inflammatory reaction. However, in mammals it has been seen only in some specific inflammations of brain.
6. Giant cells are the feature of avian inflammation and are observed in acute and chronic inflammation while in mammals these are seen only in chronic inflammation.
7. In birds, thrombocytes act as phagocytic cells.

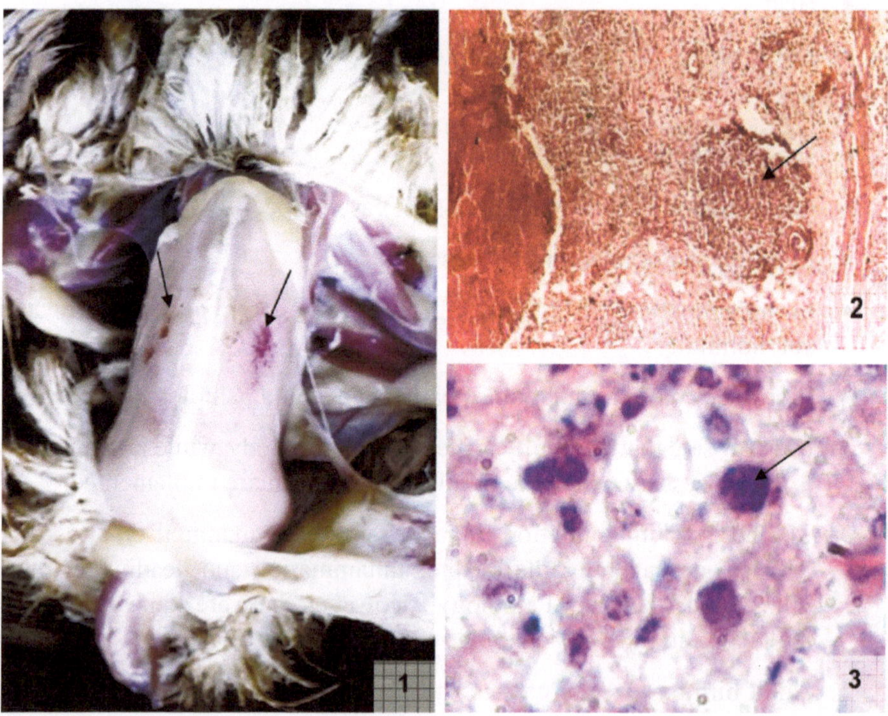

Fig. 1.1. Inflammatory reaction in poultry- **(1)** Cardinal signs of redness and swelling **(2)** Accumulation of mononuclear cells and **(3)** Presence of numerous basophils in inflammation.

8. Biphasic vascular permeability response occurs in chicken. First reaction is mediated by histamine while another reaction is mediated by unknown factors. It has been proved by treatment with antihistaminic drugs which did not stop the inflammatory reaction.

9. In chicken, inflammation caused by phytohaemagglutinin or concanavalin-A (Con-A) is characterized by skin response with infiltration of heterophils, monocytes and basophils. While in mammals, there are no neutrophils and basophils in such reactions (Fig.1.1).

2

Pathology of Nutritional Disorders

Pathology of nutritional deficiency diseases are described in chapter etiology of this book. However, specific deficiency of nutrition that leads to development of clinical signs and lesions in poultry are summarized as under (Fig.2.1 & Fig.2.2):

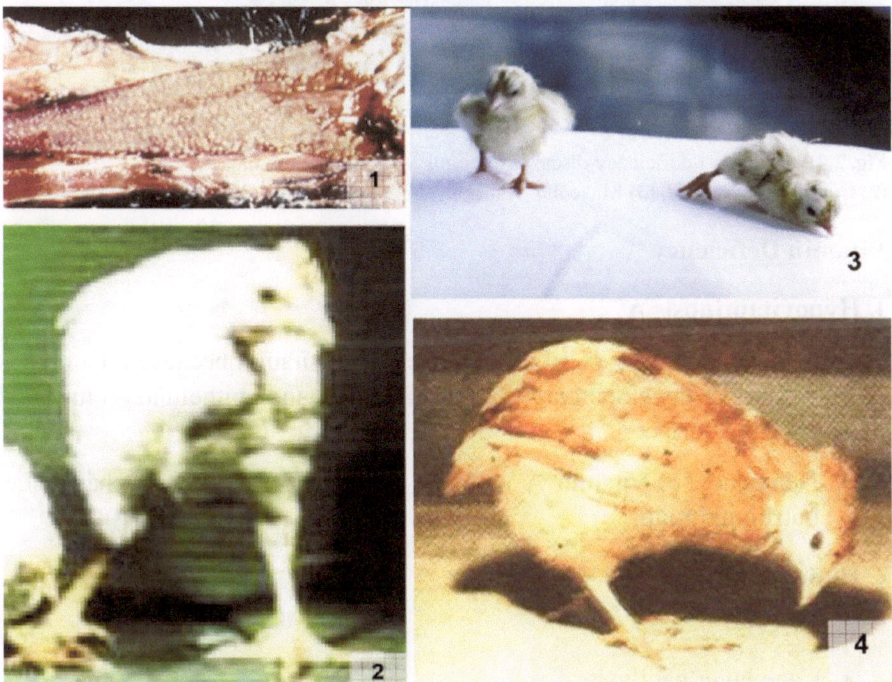

Fig. 2.1: Nutritional deficiency diseases of poultry- **(1)** Nutritional roup, **(2&3)** Rickets and **(4)** Crazy chick disease

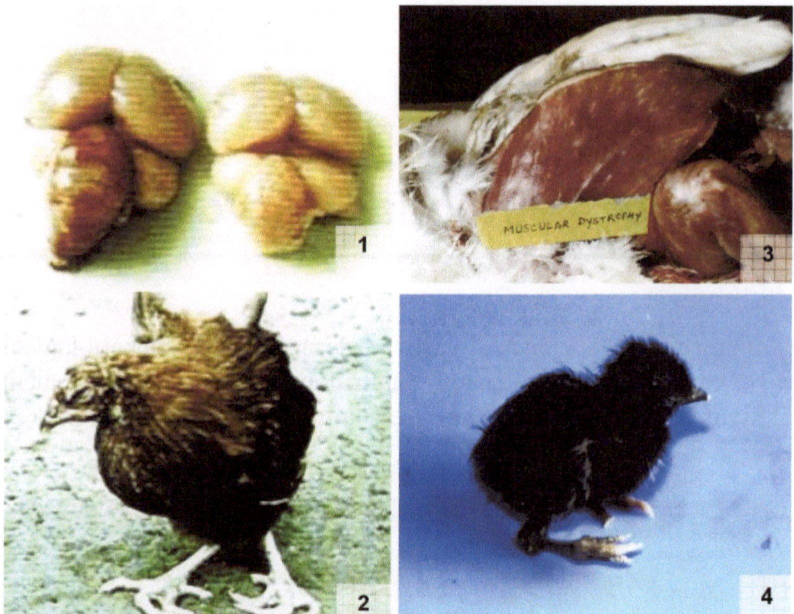

Fig. 2.2: Nutritional deficiency diseases of poultry- **(1)** Encephalomalacia, **(2)** Curled toe paralysis, **(3)** Muscular dystrophy and **(4)** Perosis in chick.

Vitamin Deficiency

1. Hypovitaminosis A

- Vitamin A is considered infection resisting vitamin because it facilitates the proper development of bursa, immunity and epithelium on mucosal and skin surfaces.
- Deficiency of vitamin A leads to swollen glands in oesophagus i.e. nutritional roup.

2. Hypovitaminosis D

- Rickets
- Cage layer paralysis
- Deformed rib junctions

3. Hypovitaminosis E

- Encephalomalacia
- Chicks push their head beneath the breast "***Crazy Chick Disease***"

- Muscular dystrophy with white necrotic areas on muscles
- Distortion of hock joint

4. Hypovitaminosis K

- Increased blood clotting time
- Blood tinged droppings
- Pale bone marrow
- Haemorrhage in breast and thigh muscles

5. Hypovitaminosis C

- Case layer fatigue

6. Hypovitaminosis B_1

- Star grazing in chicks
- Atrophy of testes
- Atrophy of ovary

7. Hypovitaminosis B_2

- Curled toe paralysis

8. Nicotinic acid/niacin deficiency

- Enlargement of joints
- Legs bend outwards

9. Pentothenic acid deficiency

- Nodular hyperplasia and cracks at foot pad.
- Scabs at commissures of the mouth; eyelids and toes
- Stunted growth
- Hypoplasia of spleen

10. Pyridoxine (B_6) deficiency

- Stunted growth
- Encephalomalacia
- Jerking movements

11. Folic acid deficiency

- Anemia
- Retardation of growth
- Perosis

12. Biotin deficiency

- Dermatitis
- Perosis
- Embryonic death
- Distorted limbs
- Big web between 3rd and 4th phalanges

13. Choline deficiency

- Perosis (Slipped tendon)
- Deformity in tibio-tarsal joint
- Fatty liver syndrome

14. Vitamin B_{12} deficiency

- Stunted growth
- Reduced hatchability
- Atrophic leg muscles
- Haemorrhage

Mineral Deficiency

1. Calcium deficiency

- Rickets
- Nodular swelling at costocondral junctions of ribs
- Bending of legs

2. Phosphorus deficiency

- Pica

3. Manganese deficiency

- Perosis
- Defective growth of bone (osteodystrophy and chondrodystrophy)
- Parrot beak

4. Zinc deficiency

- Perosis
- Scaly limb disease
- Immunosuppression

5. Copper deficiency

- Anemia
- Improper bone growth

6. Magnesium deficiency

- Stunted growth

7. Selenium deficiency

- Muscular degeneration
- Deformity in embryos (absence of beak, eye or limb)

8. Nickel deficiency

- Enlargement of hock joints

9. Iodine deficiency

- Stunted growth

10. Fluorosis/excess of fluorine

- Retarded growth
- Drop in egg production
- Deformity in bones

3

Viral Diseases

Ranikhet Disease

Ranikhet disease is a contagious viral disease of poultry characterized by high mortality petechial hemorrhage in proventriculus, ulcers and hemorrhage at caecal tonsils and pneumoencephalitis. It is also known as ***Newcastle disease*** (Fig.3.1).

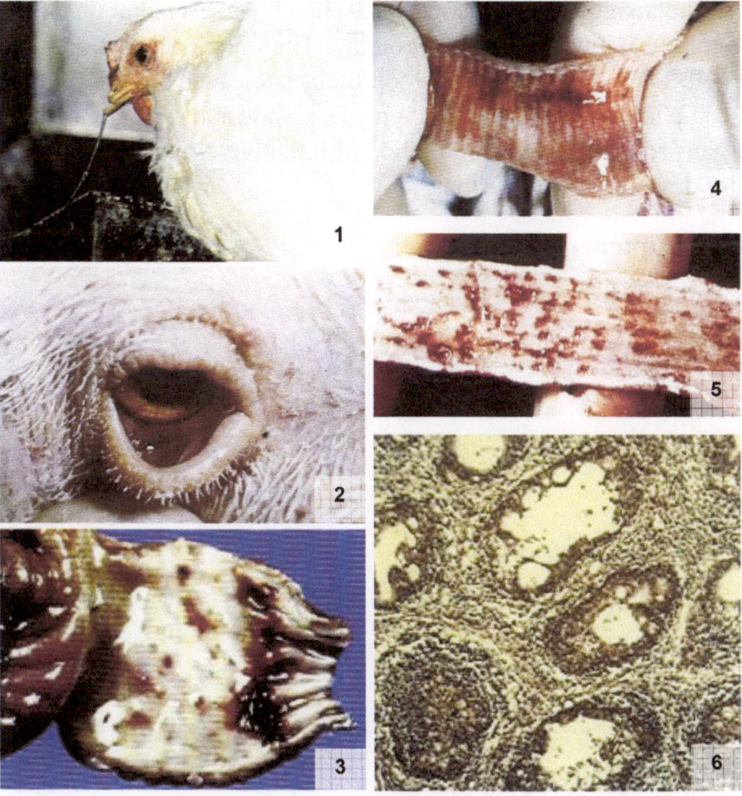

Fig. 3.1: Ranikhet disease in poultry- **(1)** Nasal discharge, **(2)** Conjunctivitis and oedema of eye lids, **(3)** Haemorrhage in proventriculus, **(4)** Haemorrhage in trachea, **(5)** Haemorrhage in intestine and **(6)** Depletion of lymphoid tissue.

Etiology

- Paramyxo virus
- RNA virus-3 types
- Lentogenic- mild virulent
- Mesogenic- moderate virulent
- Velogenic- highly virulent

Pathogenesis

The birds showing respiratory disease shed the virus in air in the form of droplets of mucus which is inhaled by susceptible birds. The virus also transmitted through ingestion of contaminated food and water and reaches in intestines where its replication occurs. The virus is attached to cells with receptors mediated by the haemagglutinin glycoprotein. Then the virus membrane fuses with cell membrane with fusion glycoproteins. Thus nucleocapsid complex enters in the cell. During replication glycoprotein is cleaved for the progeny virus particle to be infective. The virulent viruses invade and replicate in many tissues and organs resulting in the production of infective virus throughout the body and cause development of lesions.

Characteristic symptoms

- Yellowish / greenish diarrhoea
- Twitching of neck
- Heavy mortality
- Early chick mortality
- Paralysis
- Respiratory distress
- Prostration and mortality

Macroscopic features

- ***Velogenic form***
  - Petechial hemorrhage on the tip of the proventriculus papillae.
  - Hemorrhagic ulcers in intestines particularly at ileocaecal junction (caecal tonsils).

- Petechial hemorrhage on serosal surfaces of visceral organs.

•*Mesogenic form*

- Congestion of lungs and brain
- Pneumoencephalitis
- Mottling of spleen

• ***Lentogenic form***

- Hemorrhagic lesions are few or absent and low mortality.
- Drop in egg production with congestion of ovaries.

Microscopic features

- Proliferation of endothelial cells of blood vessels in brain.
- Cytoplasmic vacuolation in neurons.
- Proliferation of glial cells.
- Thrombosis in blood vessels of intestine.
- Necrosis of mucosa leading to ulcer formation in intestines specially at caecal tonsils.
- Proliferation of Kuffer cells in liver.
- Congestion in lungs.
- Congestion of ovaries and oviduct.

Diagnosis

- Symptoms and lesions
- Demonstration of antigen in brain tissue
- Immunological tests such ELISA, AGPT, CIEP for detection antigen / antibody.

Avian Influenza

Avian influenza is a highly contagious viral disease of poultry characterized by high morbidity and mortality, serofibrinosis pericarditis, air sacculitis, pneumonia, sinusitis and caseous exudate in upper respiratory tract. This disease is also known as ***fowl plague*** and occurs in pandemic form (Fig.3.2).

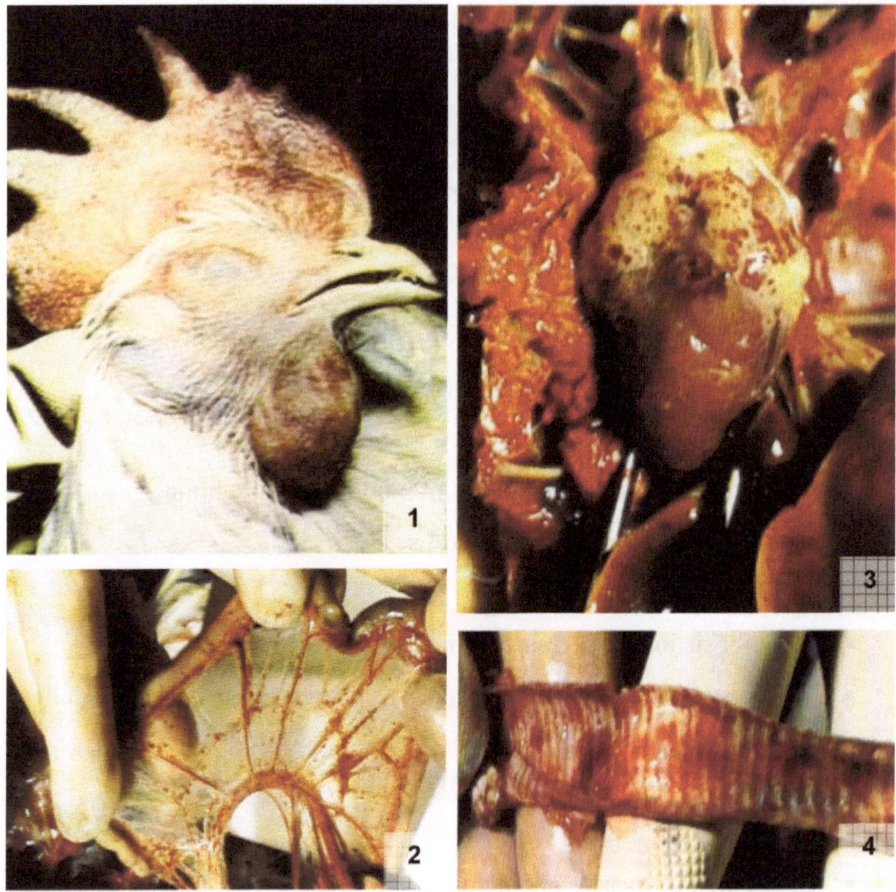

Fig. 3.2: Avian Influenza **(1)** Oedema and cyanosis in wattle, **(2)** hemorrhage in mesentery, **(3)** Hemorrhage on heart and **(4)** Haemorrhage in trachea.

Etiology

- Orthomyxovirus
- RNA virus
- Several subtypes based on Haemagglutinin (H) and Neuraminidase (N) antigens.

Pathogenesis

The source of infection is infected bird which excretes virus from respiratory tract, conjunctiva and faeces. The faecal / oral route is the main mode of transmission. The avian influenza virus adsorbs to glycoprotein receptors on the cell surface. The virus then enters in the cell by receptor mediated endocytosis. The tissue tropism of virus is involved in its pathogenicity which is receptor specific. Pathogenicity of virus is due to hemagglutinin molecule which is cleaved by host proteases and the cleaved haemagglutinin is deciding factor for viral replication and for production of infective virion particles. Due to presence of proteases the virus invades and replicates in tissues and organs resulting in generalized disease and death.

Characteristic symptoms

- Cyanosis of comb and wattle
- Oedema of face
- Respiratory distress
- Convulsions, blindness and paralysis

Macroscopic features

- Oedema of face.
- Hemorrhage on epicardium, breast muscles and inner surface of sternum.
- Necrotic foci in spleen, liver, kidneys, intestine and pancreas.
- Visceral gout and nephrosis with swollen kidneys.
- Sinusitis with caseous or mucopurulent exudate.
- Caseous exudates in air sacs.

Microscopic features

- Perivascular cuffing by lymphocytes in brain, heart, spleen and lungs.
- Coagulative necrosis in kidneys, spleen, lungs, pancreas and liver.
- Oedema in myocardium and lungs.
- Dialated tubules in kidneys with urate crystalline casts.

Diagnosis

- High morbidity and mortality.
- Symptoms and lesions
- Perivascular cuffing in brain which is absent in Ranikhet disease.
- Demonstration of H and N antigens using HA/HI test.

Marek's Disease

Marek's disease is a highly contagious disease of poultry mainly affecting young birds and characterized by thickening of nerves and malignant lymphoma in gonads and other visceral organs (Fig.3.3).

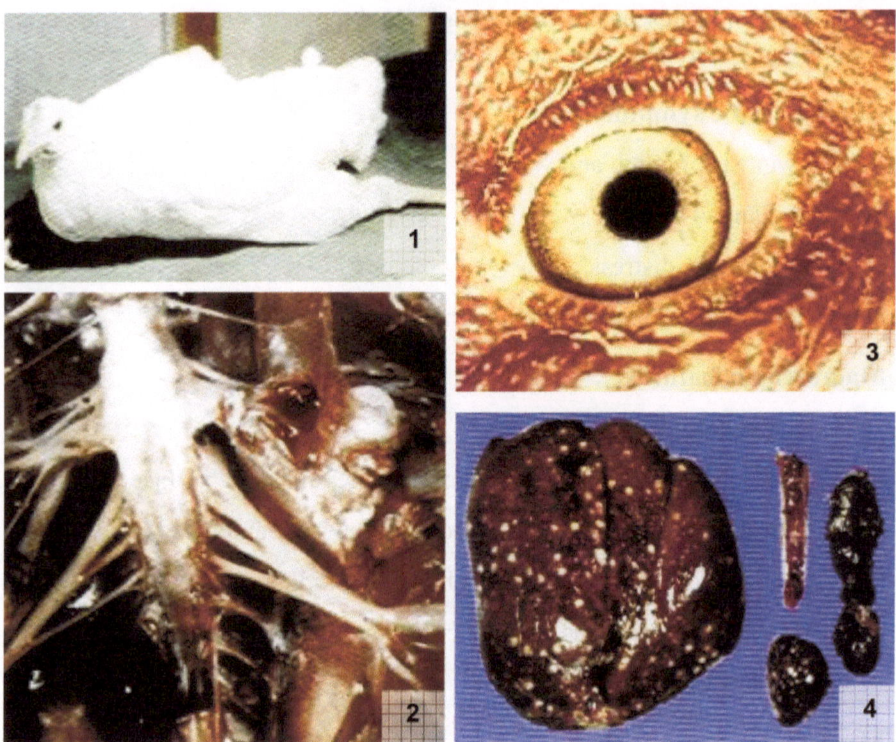

Fig. 3.3. Marek's disease in poultry- **(1)** Paralysis in bird, **(2)** Swelling of nerves, **(3)** Iridocyelitis and **(4)** Lymphoid nodules in visceral organs.

Etiology

- DNA virus
- Herpes virus
- Cell associated virus
- Produces a tumour specific antigen on the cell membrane MATSA (Marek's associated tumour surface antigen).

Pathogenesis

Feather follicle cells are the most important source of infection to the susceptible birds. However, other sources include poultry house dust and litter. Air borne spread and respiratory tract infection is most important route of infection. The virus enters through respiratory tract and it is picked up by the phagocytic cells that leads to four phase of infection.

- ***Early productive*** infection causes mainly degenerative changes i.e. cytolytic changes.
- ***Latent infection*** which coincides with the development of immune responses. Mostly T-cell are infected in latency although B-cells may also involved.
- ***Second-phase*** of cytolytic productive restrictive infection coinciding with permanent immunosuppression.
- ***Proliferative phase*** involving non-productively infected lymphoid cells which may progress to lymphoma formation. The lymphoproliferative changes constitute the final responses and may progress to tumour development.

Characteristic symptoms

- Lameness, paralysis and hanging wings
- Torticollis
- Head turns upside down
- Tumours on skin

Macroscopic features

- Thickening of nerves (Sciatic, brachial, vagus) with loss of cross striations.
- Tumours of malignant lymphoma in ovary/testes, liver, spleen, lungs, muscles, heart, kidneys, proventriculus and intestines.
- Tumours on skin.

Microscopic features

- Lymphocytic infilteration in nerves.
- Lymphofollicular reaction in visceral organs like gonads, liver, spleen, lungs and heart.
- Lymphocytes are immature and pleomorphic showing characteristic anaplastic changes.

Diagnosis

- Symptoms and lesions
- Sexually immature birds mostly affected
- Demonstration of MATSA in cells
- AGPT using feather follicles as source of viral antigen.

Avian Leucosis

Avian leucosis is a cancerous viral disease of poultry characterized by tumourous growth of blood cells in liver, spleen, lungs, ovary, kidneys and other visceral organs. Disease occurs sporadically in adult birds also known as ***big liver disease*** (Fig.3.4).

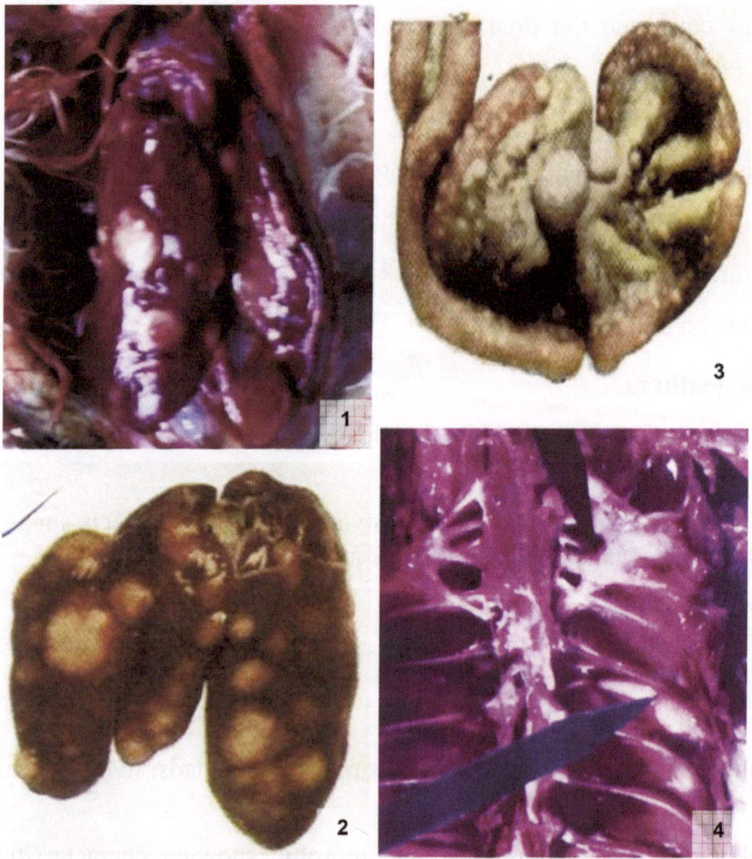

Fig. 3.4: Avian leucosis in poultry- **(1&2)** Lymphoid nodules on liver, **(3)** Lymphoid nodules on intestine and **(4)** Osteopetrosis.

Etiology

- Avian leucosis virus is a RNA virus of retroviridae family
- Virus has reverse transcriptase enzyme to convert viral RNA to DNA which incorporated in cellular DNA.

Pathogenesis

The avian leucosis virus is transmitted vertically from hen to chicks through eggs as well as horizontally through direct and indirect contact. It is a malignancy of the bursa-dependent lymphoid system. The target cells are transformed in the bursa of most birds, only few birds develop lymphoid leucosis most of tumours regress and only few enlarges and their cells enter into vascular system and produce metastatic foci in other visceral organs.

Characteristic symptoms

- Pale comb
- Enlarged abdomen
- Profuse haemorrhage from feather follicles
- Boot like appearance of shank

Macroscopic features

- Avian leucosis complex includes:

a) ***Lymphoid leucosis***

- Tumours of lymphoblasts in liver, spleen, ovary and other organs.
- Tumours are white/grey, raised and glistening.

b) ***Erythrdblastosis***

- Immature erythrocytes in blood stream, bone marrow and liver.
- Bone marrow hypertrophied and becomes cherry red in colour.

c) ***Myeloblastosis***

- Neoplastic growth of granulocytes in liver, spleen and other organs.

d) ***Osteopetrosis***

- Thickening of the long bones, limbs and ribs due to overgrowth.

Microscopic features

- Anaplastic blood cells.
- Malignant cells with mitotic figures.

Diagnosis

- Symptoms and lesions
- Big liver size with tumours.
- Sporadic occurrence in adult birds.
- Histopathological examination of affected tissue.

Infectious Bursal Disease

Infectious bursal disease is an immunosuppressive disease of birds caused by birna virus and characterized by lesions in bursa of Fabricious, lack of B-lymphocytes, deposition of urates in kidneys and ureter and hemorrhagic myositis. Morbidity rate is as high as 100% and mortality is up to 80% (Fig.3.5).

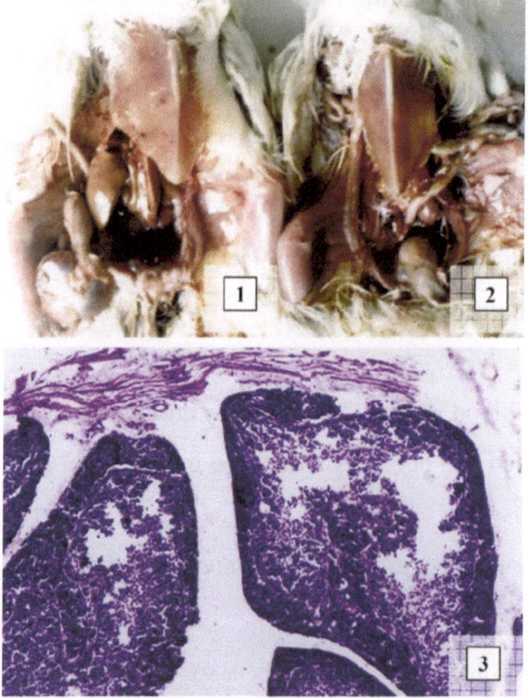

Fig. 3.5: Infectious bursal disease in poultry- **(1)** Oedema of bursa of Fabricious, **(2)** Haemorrhage in bursa of Fabricious and **(3)** Depletion of lymphoid cells from bursal follicles.

Etiology

- Birna virus
- Double stranded RNA virus having two segments.
- 5 serotypes in India.
- Very stable at 60°C for 30 min.

Pathogenesis

The virus is transmitted through contaminated feed, water and droppings of the infected birds. Most common route of infection is oral route but conjunctival and respiratory routes are also important. The incubation period is 2-3 days. After infection, within hours virus is found in macrophages and lymphoid cells in the caeca, duodenum, jejunum and Kupffer cells of the liver. The virus first reaches the liver then enters in the blood stream and distributed to different tissues including bursa. There is development of viraemia. The virus causes destruction of affected lymphoid cells (mainly B- cells and their precursors) in the bursa of Fabricious, spleen and caecal tonsils. Bursal depletion in early life may result in impaired immune responses which causes immunosuppression leading to lowered resistance to diseases.

Characteristic symptoms

- Symptoms vary due to immunosuppression
- Trembling of body
- Picking of vent
- Watery diarrhoea
- Prostration

Macroscopic features

- Enlargement of bursa of Fabricious.
- Gelatinous exudate around bursa.
- Hemorrhage in bursa giving it a blackish brown colour.
- Atrophy of bursa after 5-7 days of infection.
- Urates on kidneys and in ureter with swelling.
- Echymotic hemorrhage in muscles of thigh or breast region.
- Spleen may become swollen and later on atrophied.
- May show lesions of other diseases due to immunosuppression.

Microscopic features

- Depletion of lymphocytes in bursal follicles.
- Oedema, congestion and hemorrhage in bursa.
- Hyperplasia and vacuolar degeneration of bursal epithelial cells.
- Proliferation of fibrous tissue.
- Eosinophilic casts in tubular lumen in kidneys.
- Oedema, congestion, hemorrhage in muscles with necrosis.

Diagnosis

- Symptoms and lesions
- Immunodiagnostic tests such as AGPT, ELISA for detection of antigen / antibody.
- Isolation and identification of virus.

Infectious Bronchitis

Infectious bronchitis is a viral disease of poultry caused by corona virus and characterized by sneezing, coughing, respiratory rales, cheesy exudates in bronchi, affections of ovary and oviduct and deposition of urates in kidneys (Fig.3.6).

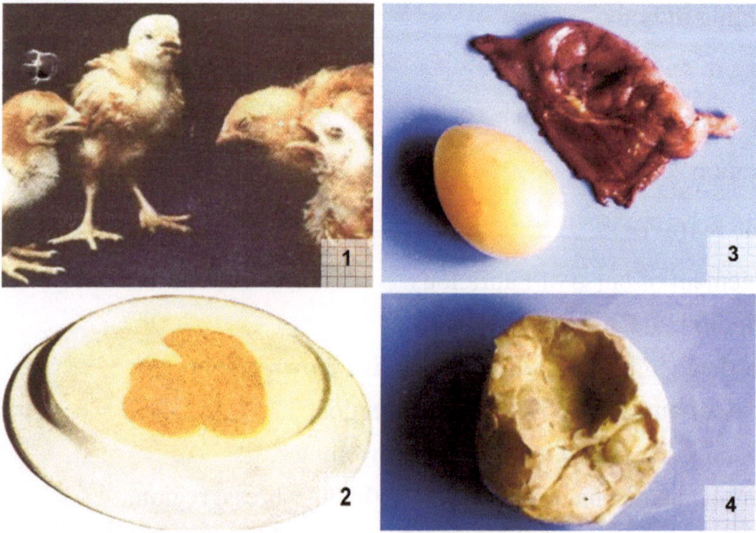

Fig. 3.6: Infectious bronchitis in poultry- **(1)** Gasping in chicks, **(2)** Thin albumin in egg, **(3)** Thin shelled eggs and salpingitis and **(4)** Deformed egg.

Etiology

- RNA virus belongs to coronaviridae family.
- Very fragile, 100 nm diameter
- May be complicated by Mycoplasma, *E.coli*, adenovirus and/or reovirus

Pathogenesis

The virus is transmitted through inhalation and also through direct contact from bird to bird. The incubation period of IB is 18-36 hours. After entering through airborne route, virus replicates in trachea and lungs and causes viraemia. Through blood stream, it reaches to various organs like kidneys, oviduct etc where it replicates and causes damage of kidney tubules which leads to reduced absorption of water, glucose and electrolytes causing dehydration and acidosis.

Characteristic symptoms

- Sneezing, coughing, respiratory rales and dyspnoea
- Drop in egg production
- Thin shelled eggs
- Thin and watery yolk

Macroscopic features

- Catarrhal or cheesy exudates in trachea, bronchi.
- Gaseous plugs in bronchi where it enters in lungs.
- Cystic dilation of oviduct.
- Ova may rupture with thin, watery albumin and yolk.
- Enlarged kidneys with deposits of urates, ureters distended due to urates.
- Stones in kidneys in layers.

Microscopic features

- Hyperplasia of epithelium in trachea.
- Congestion, haemorrhage, oedema and lymphocytic infilteration in mucosa of trachea and bronchi with necrosis and desquamation of mucosal epithelium.

- Focal accumulation of lymphocytes in oviduct and kidneys.
- Lymphoid depletion in bursa.

Diagnosis

- Symptoms and lesions
- Immunological tests to demonstrate antigen in tissue/antibody in serum
- Isolation and identification of virus

Infectious Laryngotracheitis

Infectious laryngotracheitis is a viral disease of poultry caused by herpes virus and characterized by gasping, blood tinged nasal discharge, hemorrhage in trachea and deposition of cheesy exudates in larynx and trachea. The disease mostly occurs in adult birds (Fig. 3.7).

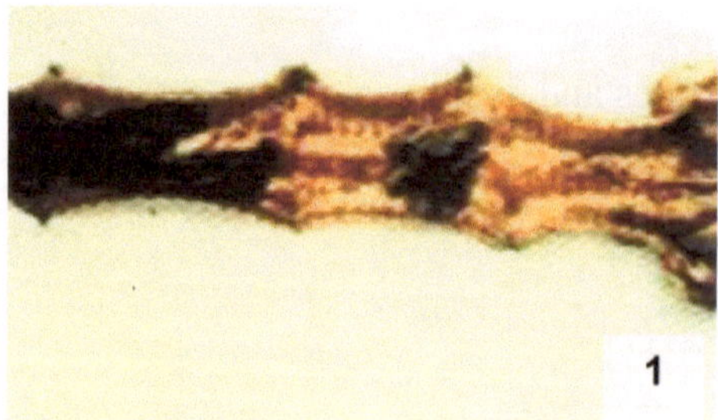

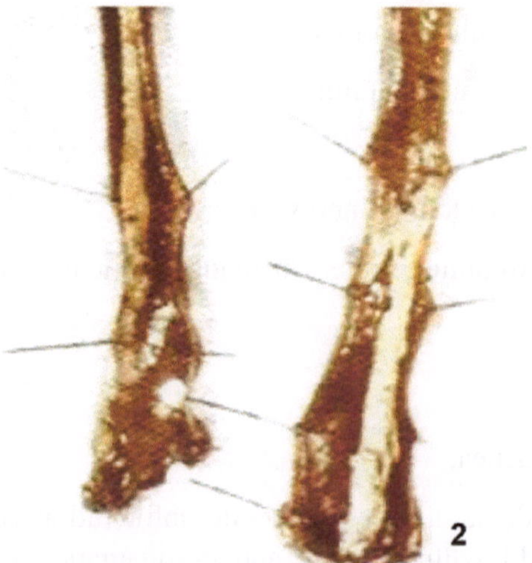

Fig. 3.7: Infectious laryngotracheitis in poultry- **(1)** Haemorrhage in trachea and **(2)** Deposition of cheesy material in trachea.

Etiology

- DNA virus belongs to herpes virus group.
- Carrier birds may excrete virus in faeces for several months.

Pathogenesis

The disease is transmitted through ingestion and inhalation. The incubation period of disease is 6-12 days. After infection, the virus intensely replicates in upper respiratory tract without viraemia. After 4-7 days of exposure virus goes to trigeminal ganglion from tracheal exposures and remains in latency. After long period activation of latent virus may occur.

Characteristic symptoms

- Watery fluid from eyes
- Dyspnoea
- Sneezing, coughing and rales
- Gasping

Macroscopic features

- Blood tinged exudate in nostrils.
- Cheesy exudate forming plugs in trachea and larynx.
- Hemorrhage in trachea.
- Conjunctivitis and swelling of intra orbital sinus.
- Bird may become blind.

Microscopic features

- Necrosis and desquamation of epithelium in tracheal mucosa with congestion and hemorrhage.
- Infiltration of lymphocytes in mucosa of trachea.
- Presence of eosinophilic intranuclear inclusions in tracheal epithelium.

Diagnosis

- Symptoms and lesions
- Tracheal impression smear may show inclusions in epithelial cells.
- Immunodiagnostic test to demonstrate antigen or antibody.

Reovirus Infection

1. Tenosynovitis (viral arthritis)

Tenosynovitis is a disease of adult birds of heavy breeds or parent stock caused by reovirus and characterized by swelling of hock joints, lameness and high morbidity with low mortality (Fig.3.8).

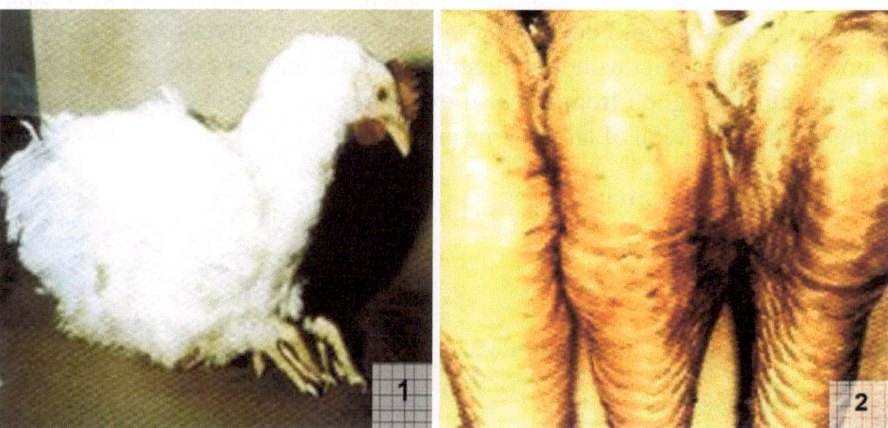

Fig. 3.8: Tenosynovitis in adult poultry- **(1)** Lameness and **(2)** Enlargement of hock joint due to rupture of gastronomies muscle tendon.

Etiology

- Reovirus, double stranded RNA virus with segmented genome having 10 segments.
- Very stable virus.
- May pass from parents to chicks through vertical transmission.

Pathogenesis

After oral infection, the virus settles in joints of the birds. It causes swelling of joint due inflammatory reaction and rupture of gastrocnemius muscle tendon.

Characteristic symptoms

- Lameness
- Swelling of hock joint
- Rupture of gastrocnemius tendon

Macroscopic features

- Swelling of hock joints and foot pads.
- Swelling of synovial sheath of tendons.
- Rupture of gastrocnemius tendon.
- Purulent or caseous exudate in joint

Microscopic features

- Epithelial hyperplasia in synovial sheaths.
- Follicular infilteration of lymphocytes.
- Ulcers on articular surface of joint.

Diagnosis

- Symptoms and lesions
- Demonstration of antigen in tendon/ synovial cells.
- Antibody in serum using immunodiagnostic tests.
- Isolation and identification of virus

2. Avian Stunting Syndrome

Avian stunting syndrome is a disease of birds affecting mainly broilers at the age of 2-4 week and characterized by low weight gain, pasty vent, and atrophy of pancreas (Fig.3.9).

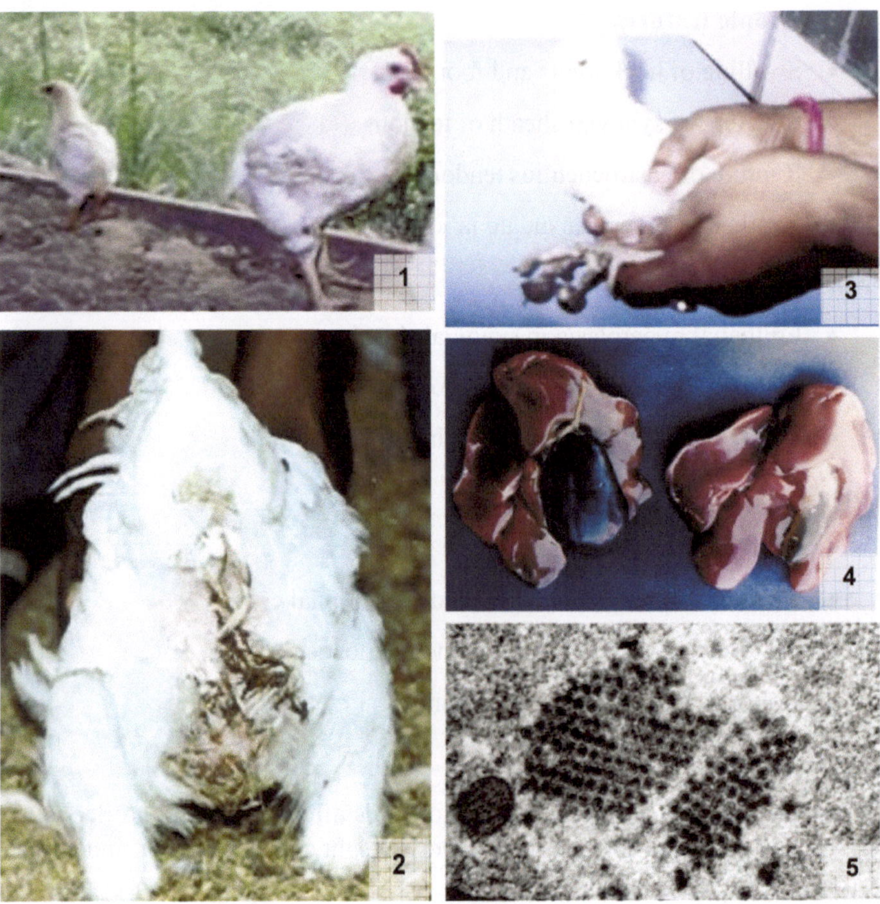

Fig. 3.9: Avian stunting syndrome in poultry- **(1)** Reduction in size of birds, **(2)** Enlargement of gall bladder, **(3)** Faecal matter on claws, **(4)** Pasty vent and **(5)** Electronphotomicrograph of avian reovirus.

Etiology

- Reovirus- double stranded RNA virus
- Very stable virus

Pathogenesis

After oral infection, the lesions are most pronounced in the mid jejunum. In enterocytes, small virion particles are detected in the villous epithelial cells. Virus causes necrosis of enterocytes and there is marked infiltration of macrophages and lymphocytes into the villi. Then through macrophages, virus spreads to lamina propria surrounding crypts and multiplication of virus causes necrosis and loss of crypts. There is villous atrophy leading to impaired digestion, poor growth and poor feathering. It also affects the pancreas causing fibrosis and atrophy.

Characteristic symptoms

- Diarrhoea
- Soiling of cloaca with semisolid cement like cheesy material '***Pasty vent***'
- Stunted growth of birds

Macroscopic features

- Stunting of the birds, low weight in about 20-50 % of the birds
- Pasty cement like grey coloured deposition on and around vent.
- Undigested food material in intestine with catarrhal enteritis
- Greenish discolouration of liver with distension of gall bladder.
- Pancreas becomes atrophied.

Microscopic features

- Necrosis and desquamation of villus epithelial cells in small intestines.
- Necrosis of pancreatic islands and proliferation of fibrous tissue.
- Infilteration of lymphocytes in intestine, pancreas, liver and gall bladder.

Diagnosis

- Symptoms and lesions
- Immunodiagnostic tests to demonstrate antigen in intestinal and pancreatic tissues.
- Isolation and identification of virus

Viral Nephritis

Viral nephritis is caused by an enterovirus characterized by nephropathy deposition of urates, lymphofollicular reaction and poor growth in broilers particularly at the age of 1-4 weeks. It is also known as ***baby chick nephropathy***.

Etiology

- RNA virus belongs to entero virus of picornaviridae family.
- Two serotypes

Pathogenesis

The disease is transmitted through ingestion of faeces contaminated materials and eggs. After ingestion, virus is detected in faeces within 2 days and maximum shedding occurs at 4-5 days. Virus is widely distributed with maximum titers in kidneys and jejunum and lower titers in bursa of Fabricious, spleen and liver. The lesions develop only in young chickens kidneys.

Characteristic symptoms

- Stunted growth of birds
- Soiling of cloaca with semisolid cheesy material and urates
- Early chick mortality

Macroscopic features

- Deposition of urates in kidneys with their swelling
- Urates deposition on visceral organs
- Poor growth of the birds
- Catarrhal enteritis

Microscopic features

- Interstitial nephritis with lymphofollicular reaction.
- Protein casts in tubules.
- Increased number of goblet cells in intestines.

Diagnosis

- Symptoms and lesions
- Demonstration of virus in intestinal epithelium and kidney tubules using immunodiagnostic tests.
- Detection of antibodies in serum
- Isolation and identification of virus

Avian Encephalomyelitis

Avian encephalomyelitis is a disease of chicks caused by a picornavirus and characterized by muscle tremors, blindness, incoordination of movements, grayish spots in muscles of gizzard and proventriculus and proliferation of microglial cells in brain. It is also known as ***epidemic tremors*** and occurs as an egg borne disease (Fig.3.10).

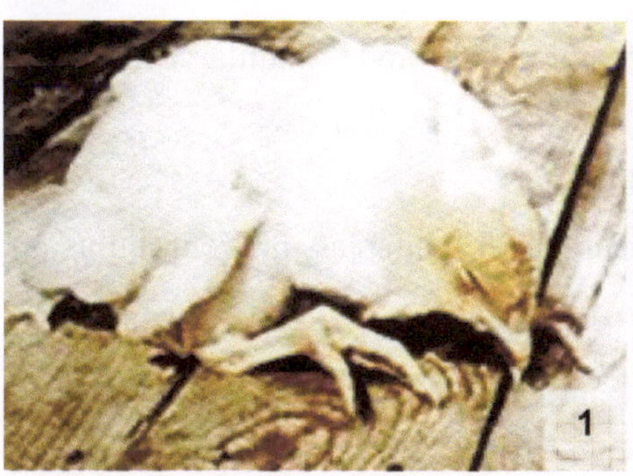

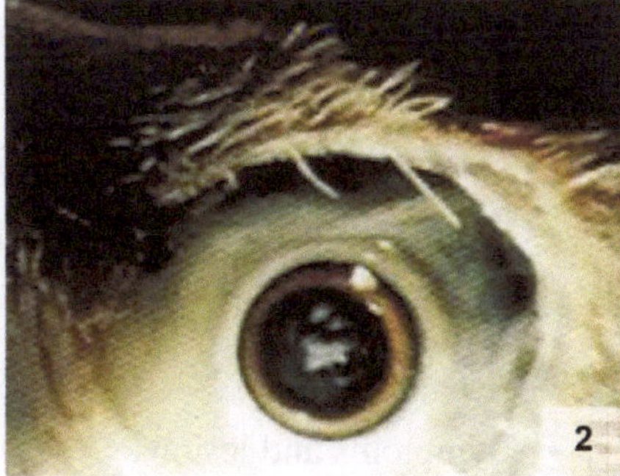

Fig. 3.10: Avian encephalomyelitis in poultry- **(1)** Paralysis of muscles and **(2)** Opacity due to cataract.

Etiology

- RNA virus of enterovirus group in picornaviridae family.
- Affinity to nervous system.
- Only one serotype.

Pathogenesis

The virus enters through ingestion of faeces contaminated feed and water. It enters in duodenal mucosa and causes viraemia. Then the virus settles in different organs like pancreas, liver, heart, kidneys, muscle, brain and spleen. The virus multiplies in perkinje cells and cerebellum and produces lesions.

Characteristic symptoms

- Tremors of muscles of head and neck.
- Paralysis leading to torticollis.
- Opacity leading to blindness.
- Morality 10-50%.

Macroscopic features

- Grayish spots in muscle of gizzard and proventriculus.
- No characteristic gross lesion.

Microscopic features

- Swelling of neurons.
- Neuronal degeneration, chromatolysis and nodular microglial proliferation.
- Perivascular lymphocytic cuffing.
- Lymphofollicular reaction in heart, liver, pancreas, proventriculus and gizzard.

Diagnosis

- Symptoms and lesions
- Demonstration of antigen/antibody using immunodiagnostic tests.
- Isolation and identification of virus

Rotaviral Diarrhoea

Rotaviral diarrhoea occurs in young birds and characterized by dehydration, enteritis and poor growth of the birds.

Etiology

- Rotavirus (serotype-7)
- Double stranded RNA virus with segmented genome (11 segments)
- Not related of mammalian rotavirus.

Pathogenesis

The virus in transmitted through faeces of infected birds through direct or indirect contact. Rotavirus infection is mainly confined to intestinal tract. The virus multiplies in the mature villus epithelial cells of small intestine. The infected epithelial cells are destroyed, resulting in villus atrophy and compensatory crypt hypertrophy. There is replacement of mature cells by immature cells deficient in digestive enzymes and in their ability to transport water and electrolytes leading to maldigestion, malabsorption and diarrhoea.

Characteristic symptoms

- Diarrhoea in chicks at 1-2 weeks of age.
- Dehydration and mortality in 5-10% birds.
- Reduced growth.

Macroscopic features

- Catarrhal, enteritis with undigested food material in intestines.
- Atrophy of bursa.
- Intestine and caeca contain fluid and gas.
- Cracking of feet /digits with feacal crusts.

Microscopic features

- Reduction in size of villi with necrosis and desquamation of mucosal villus epithelial cells.
- Infiltration of lymphocytes and mononuclear cells in intestinal mucosa.

Diagnosis

- Symptoms and lesions
- Demonstration of antigen in intestinal tissue
- Isolation and identification of virus

Avian Pox

Avian pox is a viral disease of poultry caused by a DNA virus of pox group and characterized by appearance of characteristic pock lesions on feather less parts of the body (Fig.3.11).

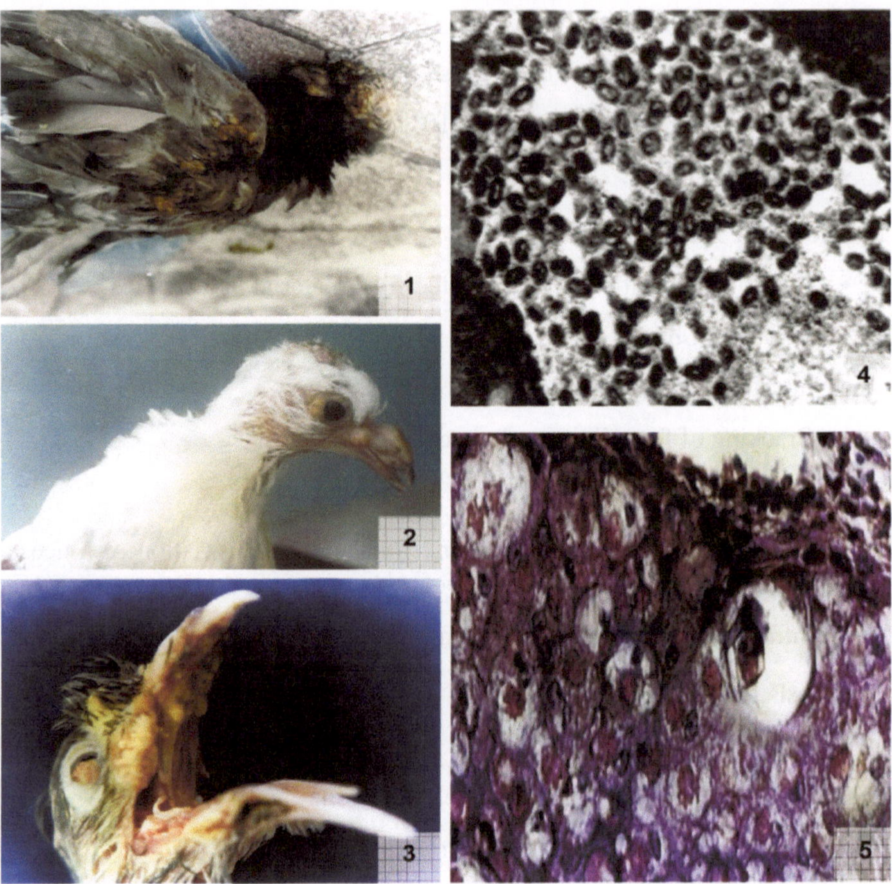

Fig. 3.11: Avian pox- **(1)** Pock lesions on back of bird, **(2)** Pock lesions on beak and eyes of bird, **(3)** Pock lesions in oral cavity, **(4)** Electronphotomicrograph of avian pox virus and **(5)** Intracytoplasmic inclusions.

Etiology

- Pox virus
- Four serotypes fowl pox, canary pox, pigeon pox, turkey pox,
- Produces pock lesions on CAM of chick embryo

Pathogenesis

The virus is transmitted through direct contact. A break in the skin is required for the virus to enter the epithelial cells. The cells of mucosa of the upper respiratory tract and mouth is highly susceptible for virus. After entering in epithelial cells, it spreads from cell to cell which is helped by production of epidermal growth factor causing proliferation of cells. Some virus enters in blood circulation and causes viraemia. Through circulation it reaches to certain organs like spleen and liver. In epithelium of skin, it produces pock lesions.

Characteristic symptoms

- Nodules on feather less parts of body *i.e.* comb, wattle and face
- Yellowish cheese like material in buccal cavity
- Swelling of eyelid leading to blindness

Macroscopic features

- Cutaneous form characterized by papule and scab on comb, wattle, face and other feather less parts of body.
- Yellowish nodules later on becomes blackish.
- In diphtheritic form, there is yellowish cheese like material on tongue, palate, laryngeal orifice.

Microscopic features

- Proliferation of epithelium in stratum spinosum layer of epidermis
- Cells show hydropic degeneration.
- Presence of intra cytoplasmic eosinophilic inclusions in cells of epidermis.

Diagnosis

- Symptoms and lesions
- Demonstration of virus inclusions in skin epithelium.
- Immunodiagnostic tests for demonstration of antigen / antibody.

Inclusion Body Hepatitis (IBH)

Inclusion body hepatitis is caused by adenovirus and characterized by anemia, necrotic and hemorrhagic lesions in liver and hemorrhage in muscles. It affects mainly growers with a mortality of about 30%. It occurs due to stress or immunosuppression in birds (Fig.3.12).

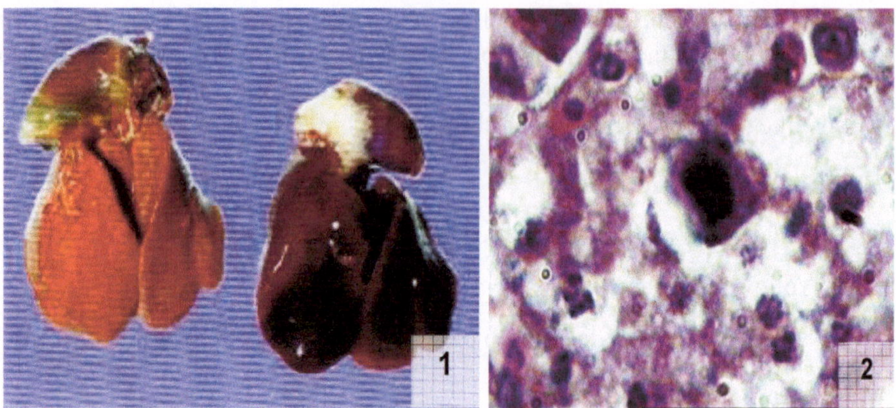

Fig. 3.12: Inclusion body hepatitis in poultry- **(1)** Congestion in liver, **(2)** Intranuclear basophilic inclusions in hepatocytes.

Etiology

- Aviadenovirus
- DNA virus of aviadenovirus group
- Quite resistant virus and found in all poultry rearing areas.

Pathogenesis

Not known. However, virus produces basophilic and eosinophilic intranuclear inclusion bodies in hepatocytes.

Characteristic symptoms

- Anemia
- Sudden mortality

Macroscopic features

- Muscles and bone marrow become pale and anemic.
- Swollen and mottled liver with petechiae and necrotic foci.
- Atrophy of bursa.
- Petechiae and ecchymoses in muscles and kidneys.
- Urates in ureters.
- Hydropericardium.

Microscopic features

- Intranuclear eosinophilic or basophilic inclusion bodies with margination of nucleus in hepatocytes.
- Necrosis and lymphocytic infiltration in liver.
- Lymphofollicular reaction in trachea.
- Depletion of lymphoid cells in spleen and bursa.

Diagnosis

- Symptoms and lesions
- Demonstration of inclusions in impression smear of liver.
- Blood examination– anemia.
- Immunodiagnostic test for antigen or antibody detection.

Hydropericardium Syndrome

Hydropericardium syndrome in caused by adenovirus and characterized by watery straw colored fluid in pericardial sac, hepatitis and atrophy of lymphoid organs. Disease occurs in growers after immunosuppression or stress with 5-10% mortality (Fig.3.13).

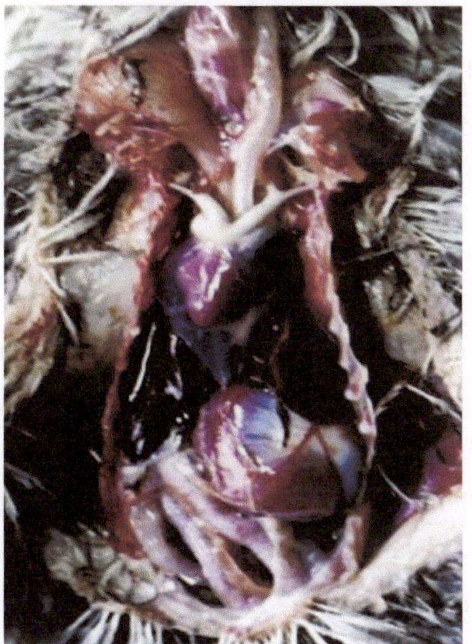

Fig. 3.13: Hydropericardium syndrome in poultry.

Etiology

- Aviadenovirus
- DNA virus
- Present in poultry house environment
- Quite resistant virus
- Affects birds after stress

Pathogenesis

The disease spreads through both vertical and horizontal transmission. In breeding stocks, virus may remain in latent phase until onset of maturity and sheds when there is immunosuppresion or stress. The virus multiplies in intestine and through circulation reaches in various organs including pericardium and produces lesions.

Characteristic symptoms

- Enlargement of abdomen
- Anemia
- Sudden mortality

Macroscopic features

- Straw colored fluid in pericardial sac (8-10 ml fluid).
- Atrophy of heart with petechiae on myocardium.
- Haemorrhagic and necrotic foci in liver.
- Atrophy of bursa and spleen.

Microscopic features

- Haemorrhage in myocardium, increased distance in myofibrils due to oedema.
- Degenerative changes in myofibrils.
- Intranuclear eosinophilic or basophilic inclusions in liver cells
- Infiltration of lymphocytes in liver, heart and kidneys
- Lymphoid depletion in spleen and bursa.

Diagnosis

- Symptoms and lesions
- Fluid in pericardial sac
- Isolation and identification of virus
- Immunodiagnostic tests for detection of antigen of antibody.

Egg Drop Syndrome

Egg drop syndrome occurs in adult laying birds caused by adenovirus and characterized by decrease in egg production, oedema in oviduct and splenomegaly(Fig.3.14).

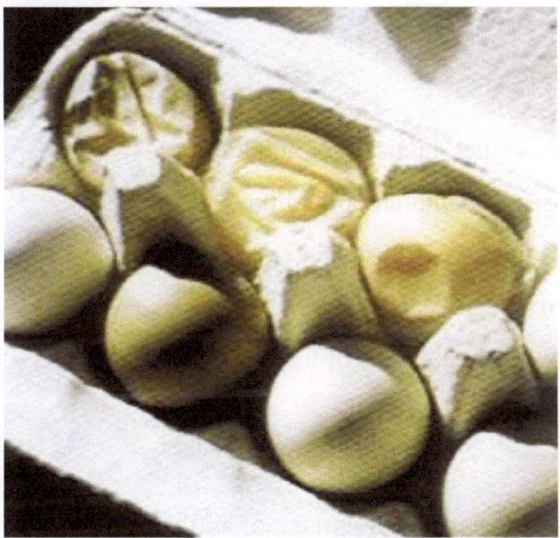

Fig. 3.14: Egg trop syndrome in poultry- Thin shelled abnormal eggs.

Etiology

- Aviadenovirus
- DNA virus

Pathogenesis

The disease is mainly transmitted through vertical transmission. After infection in laying hens, the virus grows to a limited extent in nasal mucosa followed by viraemia with replication of virus in lymphoid tissues throughout body specially in spleen and thymus. Infundibulum of oviduct is consistently affected, massive viral replication occurs in the pouch shell glands which coincides with production of thin shell eggs.

Characteristic symptoms

- Drops in production of eggs by 35- 40 percent.
- Thin shelled depigmented and cracked shelled eggs.
- Diarrhoea.

Macroscopic features

- Thin shelled, cracked or depigmented eggs.
- Oedema of oviduct, later on atrophy of oviduct.
- Splenomegaly.

Microscopic features

- Lymphoid aggregates in oviduct, lungs, liver and kidneys.
- Degeneration and necrosis of glandular epithelium.
- Hyaline changes in muscular layer of oviduct.
- Lymphoid hyperplasia in spleen.
- Intranuclear inclusions in epithelial cells of tubular glands.

Diagnosis

- Symptoms and lesions
- Immunodiagnostic tests for detection of antigen or antibody
- Isolation and identification of virus

Chicken Anemia

Chicken anemia is a viral disease of growers caused by DNA virus and characterized by watery blood, pale mucous membrane, reduced body weight and atrophy of bursa and thymus. It is also known as ***Anemia dermatitis syndrome***. Disease occurs in birds with stress or immunosuppression. It may also be transmitted in chicks through vertical transmission (Fig.3.15).

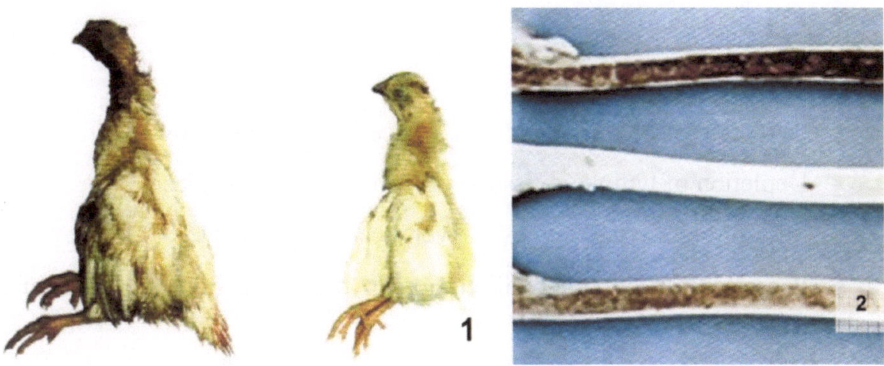

Fig. 3.15: Chicken anemia- **(1)** Healthy bone marrow and **(2&3)** Anemic bone marrow.

Etiology

- DNA virus
- Chicken anemia agent (CAA)
- Smallest virus having 24-26 nm diameter

Pathogenesis

The disease is transmitted both horizontally and vertically. In vertical transmission through hatching eggs and horizontally by direct/ indirect contact usually through oral route by ingestion of infected materials. After entering in chicks, it causes functional changes in splenic thymocytes and splenic and bone marrow macrophages. The main site of viral replication are precursor T-cells in the thymic cortex and hematoblasts in bone marrow. Destruction of these cells is responsible for immunosuppression and anemia.

Characteristic symptoms

- Pale skin and mucus membrane
- Loss of weight
- 5-10% mortality
- Thin watery blood with increased PCV

Macroscopic features

- Subcutaneous petechiae.
- Pale muscles, week emaciated carcass with reduced weight.
- Atrophy of bursa and thymus.

- Pale bone marrow.

Microscopic features

- Depletion of erythroid and myeloid cells in bone marrow.
- Depletion of lymphoid tissue in thymus, bursa and spleen.
- Infiltration of lymphocytes in liver, heart and kidneys
- Perivascular lymphoid infilteration in liver with fibrinoid thrombi in sinusoids.

Diagnosis

- Symptoms and lesions
- Immunodiagnostic tests for detection of antigen or antibody.
- Isolation and identification of virus

4

Pathology of Bacterial Diseases

Salmonellosis

Salmonellosis is caused by G-bacteria Salmonella and characterized by early chick mortality with necrosis and hemorrhage in liver, heart and spleen and enlarged bronze coloured liver with focal or diffuse necrosis, marbled spleen and/or oophoritis and salpingitis in adults (Fig.4.1).

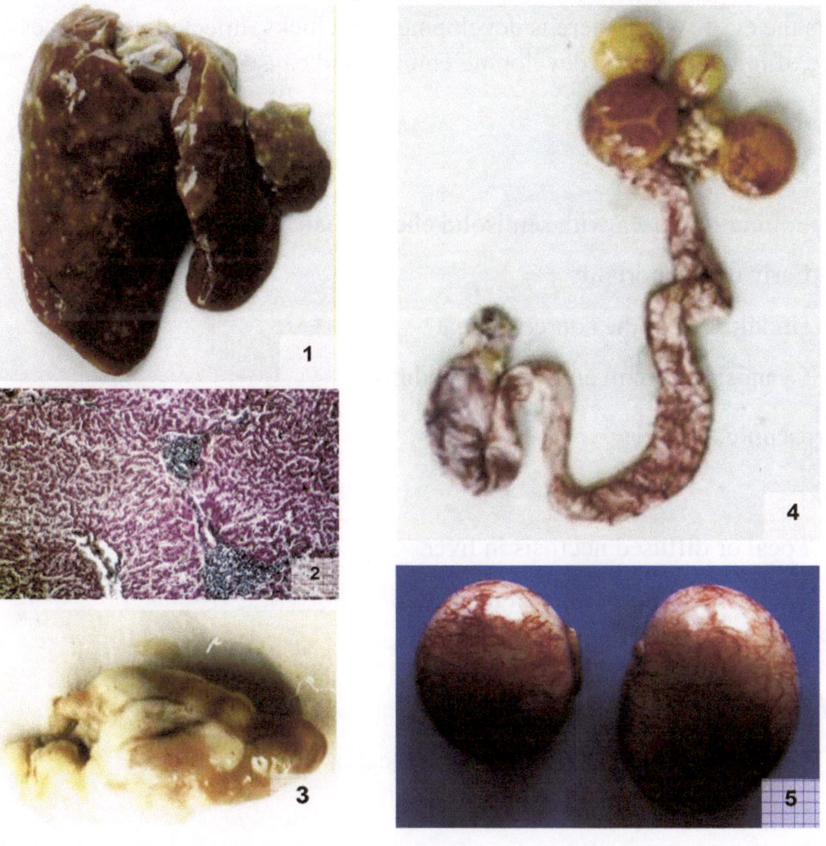

Fig. 4.1: Salmonellosis in poultry- **(1)** Focal necrosis in liver, **(2)** Microscopic features necrosis and congestion in liver, **(3)** Necrotic patches in heart, **(4)** Congestion in ovary and oviduct and **(5)** Congestion in testicles.

Etiology

- *Salmonella enteritidis* var. Galinarum *(S.* Galinarum).
- G-, rod, non lactose fermenter.
- White small colonies on MLA and pink on BGA.

Pathogenesis

The organism is transmitted horizontally through contaminated feed and water and vertically through ovary from hen to chicks. Its incubation period is generally 4-5 days. After entering through oral route, the bacteria adhere to intestinal epithelial cells, which is first step of disease occurrence; adherence occurs with type I fimbriae and a mannose resistant haemagglutinin. The virulence of organism depends on the initial degree of mucosal invasiveness and diarrhoea. In vertical transmission, the organism enters into the ovary and infects the eggs. When there is development of chicks, infected yolk serves as source of infection to the developing embryo and causes disease.

Characteristic symptoms

- Diarrhoea
- Soiling of cloaca with semisolid cheesy material
- Early chick mortality
- Huddling near the source of heat
- Cyanosis of comb and wattle in adults

Macroscopic features

Chicks

- Focal or diffused necrosis in liver.
- Semisolid cheesy material in cloaca.
- Unabsorbed yolk.

Adults

- Copper colour enlarged liver with focal or diffuse necrosis.
- Enlarged, mottled spleen.
- Catarrhal enteritis.

- Necrotic lesions on heart.
- Ovaries / testes congested.

Microscopic features

- Necrotic hepatitis
- Necrosis in myocardium with infiltration of lymphocytes, heterophils and macrophages.
- Congestion in ovary, testicles and oviduct with suppuration.
- G^- organisms demonstrable in central necrotic areas.

Diagnosis

- Symptoms and lesions
- Isolation of organism from heart blood and /or liver.
- Gram's staining of smears for demonstration of salmonella organism.

Colibacillosis

Colibacillosis is caused by *E.coli* and characterized by various syndromes like colisepticemia, air sacculitis, coligranuloma, and omphalitis in birds depending on the age and type of strain of *E.coli* involved.

Etiology

- *Escherichia coli*
- G- Coccobacilli
- Pink colony on MLA and white colony on BGA

1. Colisepticemia

Colisepticemia is a disease of young broilers due to bad management and stress and characterized by fibrinous pericarditis and hepatitis (Fig.4.2).

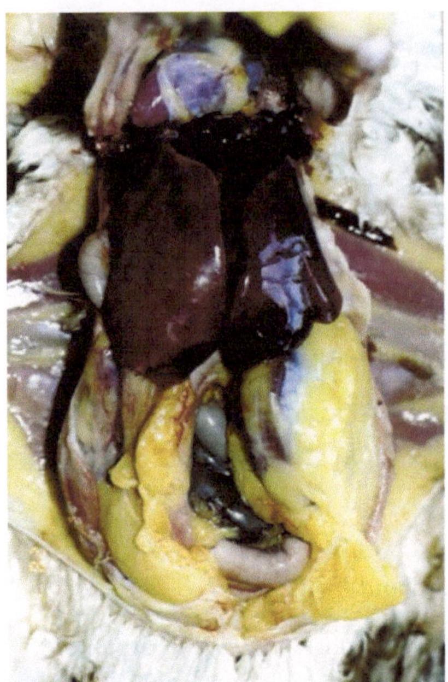

Fig. 4.2: Colisepticemia in poultry- Fibrinous hepatitis and pericarditis.

Pathogenesis

Faecal contamination of the eggs may result in the penetration of *E. coli* through the shell due to creation of negative pressure inside the eggs. This is considered most important source of infection. Bacteria may be found in the litter, dust and faecal matter. Feed is often contaminated with excreta. The bacteria is normal inhabitant in digestive tract of poultry. Birds with intact defense is resistant to *E. coli* but when defense system is compromised due to bacterial, viral, parasitic infections, toxins, poor ventilation, dust conditions etc., this infection may cause disease. Exposure to dust and ammonia results in removal of cilia of upper respiratory tract which permits the bacteria to colonize and cause respiratory infection. On entry the bacteria multiply in blood and produce septicemia.

Characteristic symptoms

- Diarrhoea
- Soiling of cloaca with semisolid cheesy material
- Dyspnoea

Macroscopic features

- Milky fluid in pericardium
- Presence of whitish pseudo membrane over pericardium.
- Fibrinous covering over liver.

Microscopic features

- Fibrinous pericarditis with infiltration of heterophils, macrophages and lymphocytes.
- Necrosis in liver with fibrinous and purulent exudate.

2. Coligranuloma (Hjarre's Disease)

Coligranuloma is a sporadic chronic disease of adult birds characterized by the presence of nodule in intestines (Fig.4.3).

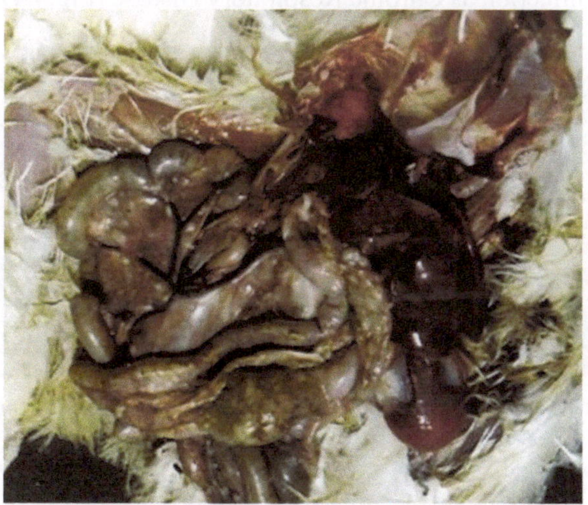

Fig. 4.3: Coligranuloma in poultry.

Pathogenesis

The bacteria enter in the intestines through penetration and settles there to cause chronic inflammation characterized by formation of nodules in intestines. These nodules are composed of cheesy material and fibrosis.

Characteristic symptoms

- Diarrhoea
- Soiling of cloaca with semisolid cheesy material

Macroscopic features

- Presence of nodules on intestine.
- Small millet size or large nodule on duodenum, caecum and liver.
- Sporadic occurrence, chronic disease seen in adults or age old birds.

Microscopic features

- Caseous necrotic area in centre covered by macrophages, lymphocytes and giant cells.
- Organisms can be demonstrated on Gram's staining in central necrotic area.

3. Air sacculitis

Air sacculitis is a disease of growers and adults and occurs along with *Mycoplasma gallisepticum* infection as Chronic Respiratory Disease (Fig.4.4).

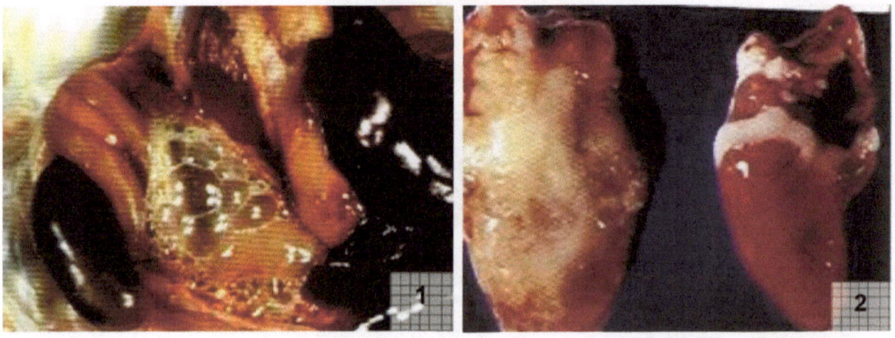

Fig. 4.4. Air sacculitis in poultry-**(1)** Cheesy material in air sacs and **(2)** Milky fluid on pericardium.

Pathogenesis

This organism is normal inhabitant of gut and is continuously excreted in droppings which contaminate the litter and environment of the poultry house. Adverse weather conditions and accumulation of ammonia and poor ventilation with dusty environment predisposes birds for *E.coli* infection as there is loss of cilia in upper respiratory tract that facilitates the entry of organisms to cause disease.

Characteristic symptoms

- Generally occurs in birds of 5-12 weeks age

- Common in overcrowded environment
- Gasping
- Dyspnoea

Macroscopic features

- Cloudiness in air sacs.
- Increased thickening of air sacs.
- Milky fluid in pericardium.

Microscopic features

- Fibrinous pericarditis.
- Suppurative air sacculitis.

4. Omphalitis

Omphalitis is a disease of newly hatched chicks and characterized by thin, watery, coagulated unabsorbed yolk (Fig.4.5).

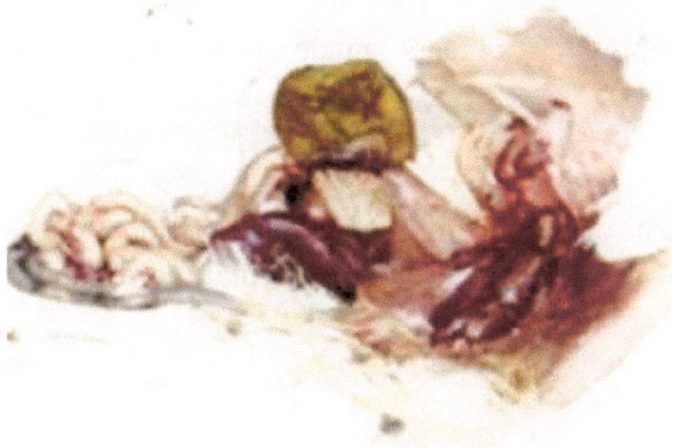

Fig. 4.5: Omphalitis in chicks.

Pathogenesis

This infection is generally associated with inflammed naval or bacteria can multiply in the hatching eggs following faecal contamination of the shell. Some other bacteria also cause yolk sac infection like staphylococcus, pseudomonas, proteus and clostridia. The bacteria rapidly multiply in the intestine of newly hatched chicks and infection spreads from chick to chick in hatchery and brooders.

Characteristic symptoms

- Sleepiness
- Aggregation near the source of heat

Macroscopic features

- Presence of unabsorbed yolk
- Yolk becomes thin and watery with precipitates
- Yolk sac membrane becomes thickened due to congestion and exudate
- Intestines congested

Microscopic features

- Focal necrotic hepatitis.
- Congestion and infiltration of heterophils in yolk sac membrane.

Diagnosis

- Symptoms and lesions
- Isolation of *E.coli* from heart blood.
- Gram's staining of impression smears made from nodules in coligranuloma.

Infectious Coryza

Infectious coryza is a disease of adult birds caused by *Haemophilus paragallinarum* and characterized by swollen head, foul smelling discharge from nostrils and eyes (Fig.4.6).

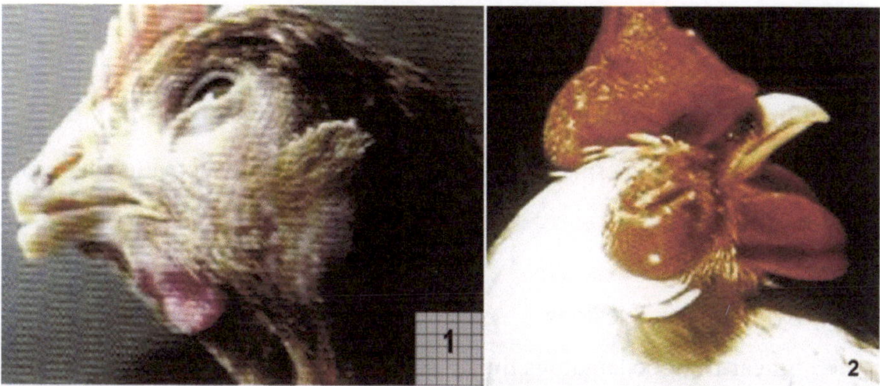

Fig. 4.6: Coryza in poultry- **(1)** Swelling of face and **(2)** Swelling of comb and conjunctivitis.

Etiology

- *Haemophilus paragallinarum.*
- G^-, bipolar, filamentous, coccoid

Pathogenesis

Source of infection is infected and carrier birds. It spreads through drinking water contaminated by nasal discharge. Airborne infection or direct contact may also play role in transmission of disease. After entry organism adhere to the ciliated mucosa of upper respiratory tract. The bacteria contain the capsule and hemagglutination antigen (HA) which play an important role in colonization. During proliferation, toxic substances are released leading to development of lesions.

Characteristic symptoms

- Discharge from nostrils and eyes
- Swollen face and wattle
- Sneezing
- Dyspnoea

Macroscopic features

- Swelling of face due to exudate in infraorbital sinuses.
- Congestion of nasal mucosa.
- Watery discharge from nostrils.

Microscopic features

- Mucopurulent exudate in trachea.
- Fibrinopurulent cellulites
- Mesothelial hyperplasia, fibrinous exudates with oedematus thickening of air sacs.

Diagnosis

- Symptoms and lesions
- Smear from oedematous fluid, stained with Gram's staining for bipolar, G^- organisms.
- Isolation from swabs taken from infraorbital sinuses.

Fowl Cholera

Fowl cholera is a contagious disease of poultry caused by *Pasteurella multocida* and characterized by cyanotic comb, swelling of wattles, fibrinous air sacculitis and pneumonia (Fig.4.7).

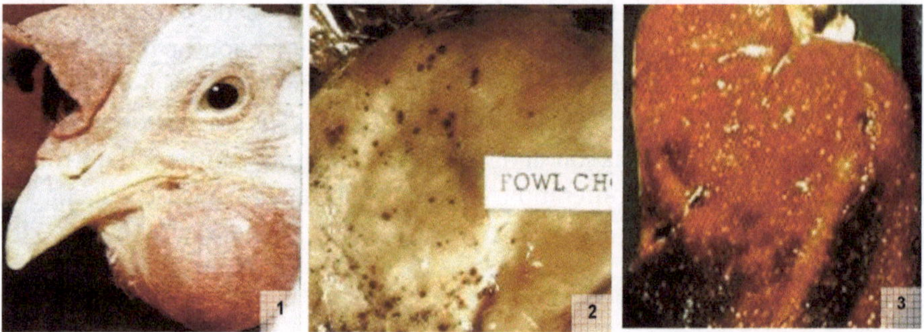

Fig. 4.7: Fowl cholera- **(1)** Swelling of wattles, **(2)** Haemorrhage on subcutaneous region and **(3)** Miliary granuloma in liver.

Etiology

- *Pasteurella multocida*
- G^-, bipolar, capsulated.

Pathogenesis

Source of infection are infected birds and rats act as reservoir. The disease mainly spreads through contaminated water and feed troughs. Birds may also be infected by oral, nasal and congenital routes. The organism enters through mucous membrane of the pharynx or upper respiratory tract. After entry organism produces sufficient quantities of endotoxin to contribute pathological processes.

Characteristic symptoms

- Cyanosis of comb and wattle
- Diarrhoea and soiling of cloaca
- Discharge from nostrils

Macroscopic features

- Bluishness of comb and oedema of wattles.
- Petechiae on heart, gizzard muscles and intestinal serosa.
- Fibrinous air sacculitis.
- Small necrotic (pinpoint size) foci on liver.

Microscopic features

- Focal area of necrosis in liver with suppuration.
- Congestion and heterophilic infiltration in lungs.
- Bipolar organisms can be demonstrated in lung and liver.

Diagnosis

- Symptoms and lesions
- Demonstration of bipolar organisms in blood smears/impression smears stained by methylene blue.
- Isolation of organisms.

Necrotic Enteritis

Necrotic enteritis is caused by clostridium, which commonly occurs after coccidiosis in chickens and characterized by necrotic patches in intestines, atrophy of spleen and breast muscles (Fig.4.8).

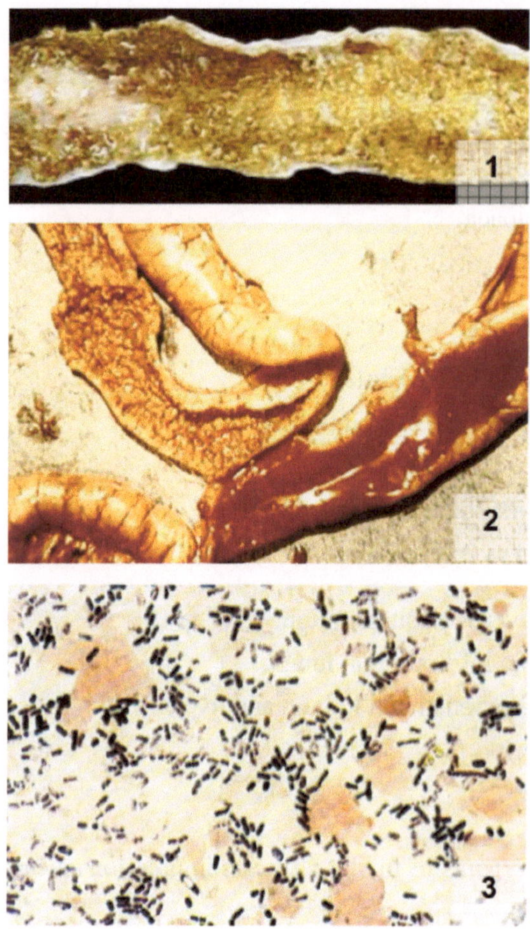

Fig. 4.8. (1&2): Necrotic enteritis due to *Clostridium* sp. and **(3)** Clostridial organism.

Etiology

- Alpha toxins of *Clostridium perfringens* type A, C, E and F.
- Intestine predisposed by coccidiosis, which provides anaerobic conditions to *Clostridium sp.* organisms.

Pathogenesis

The bacteria are present in faeces, soil, dust, contaminated feed and litter or intestinal contents. Contaminated feed or litter act as source of infection. The coccidial infection causes damage in the intestines to produce anaerobic conditions which predisposes the birds for clostridial infection. After entering through damaged intestines of the birds, the organism proliferates and liberates toxins which are responsible for intestinal mucosal necrosis.

Characteristic symptoms

- Drooling of saliva
- Emaciation in chronic cases
- Watery diarrhoea

Macroscopic features

- Yellowish brown necrotic areas involving whole small intestine.
- Small necrotic patches in liver.
- Distended gall bladder.
- Atrophy of spleen, breast muscles and testes.

Microscopic features

- Necrosis of villi of intestinal mucosa.
- Degeneration and necrosis of hepatocytes.
- Atrophy of spleen and bursa as evidenced by proliferation of connective tissue.

Diagnosis

- History- It occurs after coccidiosis
- Symptoms and lesions
- Demonstration of G^+ rods in the necrotic lesions of intestine and liver

Campylobacter Hepatitis

Campylobacter hepatitis is caused by *Campylobacter* sp. and characterized by necrotic hepatitis, hydropericardium, and catarrhal enteritis.

Etiology

- *Campylobacter jejuni*
- *C. hepaticus* and *E.coli* mixed infection
- Comma shaped, Gram negative

Pathogenesis

Transmission of disease occurs through faecal contamination of water, feed, utensils and other fomites. The organism affects the liver from where it can be isolated. It causes enlargement of liver besides necrosis and hemorrhage.

Characteristic symptoms

- Pale comb
- Drop in egg production(25-33%)

Macroscopic features

- Liver enlarged, friable with necrotic and hemorrhagic areas.
- Rupture of liver with hematoma in abdominal cavity
- Hydropericardium
- Atrophy of ovaries / testes
- Enlargement of spleen
- Pale and watery bone marrow.

Microscopic features

- Necrosis of hepatocytes and infiltration of heterophils in liver.
- Necrosis of myofibrils and hemorrhage in epicardium.
- Catarrhal enteritis.
- Comma shaped, Gram-negative organisms in liver sections and impression smears.

Diagnosis

- Demonstration of comma shaped organisms in impression smears of liver, bile and intestinal mucosa.
- Isolation of causative organisms.

Staphylococcosis

Staphylococcosis is caused by *Staphylococcus aureus* and characterized by hemorrhagic or gangrenous dermatitis, bumble foot, septicemia, arthritis and sternal bursitis (Fig.4.9).

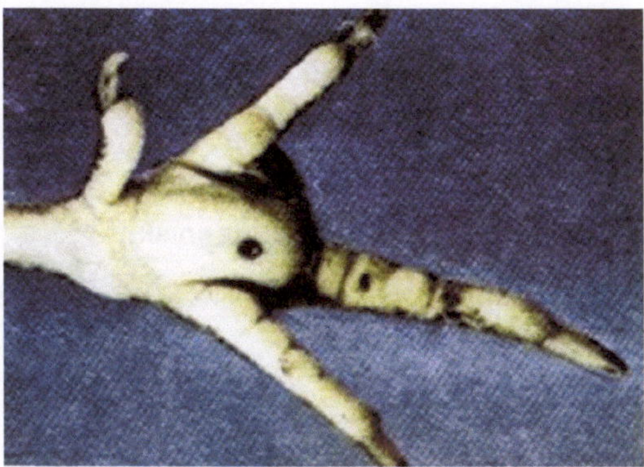

Fig. 4.9: Bumble foot in a bird

Etiology

- *Staphylococcus aureus.*
- G+, cocci, Coagulase positive.
- Toxins - enterotoxins, leucocidin and hemolysin.

Pathogenesis

The bacteria is often found in the skin, nasal passage, on beak and foot of apparently normal chickens. When there is injury in the skin or mucus membrane, it is exposed to the infection. There is formation of abscess with swelling, heat and some pain. In bumble foot the undersurface of the foot is first affected.

Characteristic symptoms

- Inflammed and hemorrhagic skin
- Formation of gangrene- greenish / blackish disclouration of skin
- Swelling of joints
- Hard swelling of foot pad with ulceration

Macroscopic features

- Dermatitis and gangrene in skin of broilers
- Bumble foot characterized by hard, fibrous swelling and ulceration of foot pad.
- Arthritis and synovitis with swelling of joints, caseous mass in joints.

- Endocarditis\
- Sternal bursa showed deposition of caseous mass.

Microscopic features

- Suppurative dermatitis with areas of gangrene formation in skin.
- Demonstration of G^+, cocci organisms in caseous mass of the tissue sections.

Diagnosis

- Symptoms and lesions
- Isolation of staphylococci.
- Demonstration of organisms in impression smears/tissue sections stained with Gram's stain.

Tuberculosis

Tuberculosis is a chronic disease of birds caused by *Mycobacterium avium* and characterized by granulomatous nodules in liver, spleen, intestines, air sacs and lungs. The disease occurs sporadically in adult birds (Fig.4.10).

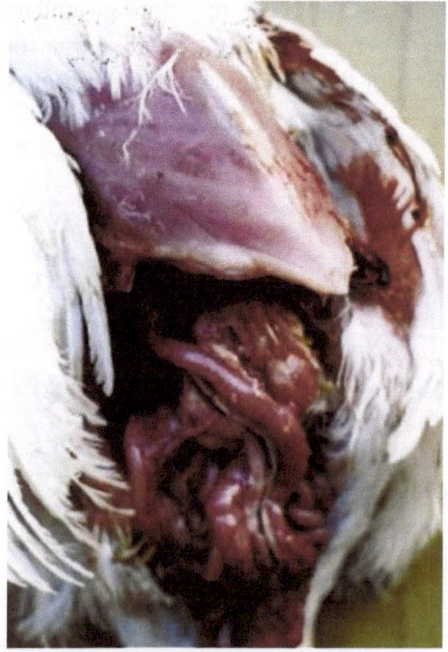

Fig. 4.10: Small tubercles in intestines.

Etiology

- *Mycobacterium avium*
- Acid fast bacilli.
- 30 serotypes, serotype 1 and 2 are pathogenic.

Pathogenesis

The most important source of infection are infected birds which shed the causative organisms in faeces. It is transmitted through ingestion of contaminated feed and water. After ingestion, it causes delayed type hypersensitivity and the activated macrophages have an increased capacity to kill the organisms. DTH reaction is mediated by lymphocytes which release lymphokines that act to attract, immobilize and activate mononuclear cells from blood at the site where virulent bacilli or their product exists. Tumour necrosis factor (TNF) alone or along with interleukin-2 (IL-2) is associated with macrophage killing of bacteria. Activated macrophages that lack sufficient microbicidal components to kill virulent tubercle bacilli are destroyed by the intracellular growth of the organisms. The toxic lipids and factors released cause disruption of the phagosome, inhibits phagolysosome formation, interfere with release of hydrolytic enzymes from the affected lysosomes or inactivate lysosomal enzymes released into the cytoplasmic vacuoles.

Characteristic symptoms

- Weakness
- Emaciation

Macroscopic features

- White, raised, dry and cheesy exudate containing nodules in liver, spleen, intestines, air sacs and lungs.
- Rupture of liver, hemorrhage and clot in abdominal cavity.

Microscopic features

- Caseative necrosis infiltrated by macrophages, lymphocytes, epithelioid and giant cells.
- This tubercle is covered by proliferation of fibroblasts.
- Acid fast bacilli in the central necrosed area

Diagnosis

- Demonstration of pea size granulomatous lesions.
- Impression smear from necrotic lesion and acid fast staining to demonstrate the acid fast bacilli.
- Tuberculin testing with avian tuberculin on skin of wattle or comb. 0.2 ml I/D tuberculin and reaction observed after 48 hrs as hot, painful swelling at the site of injection.
- Histopathological examination of affected tissue and demonstration of acid fast bacilli using special stains.

5

Path of Chlamydial Disease

Ornithosis

Ornithosis is caused by Chlamydia and characterized by enlargement of liver and spleen, serofibrinous pericarditis, air sacculitis and enteritis. This is also known as ***chlamydiosis***, ***psittacosis*** and is more common in parrots, pigeons and other psittacine birds.

Etiology

- *Chlamydia psittaci* group B
- Size 0.3 to 1.5 m
- Disease spreads from wild birds

Pathogenesis

The disease mainly spreads through inhalation of contaminated dust. After entering into body, the organism multiplies in the lungs, air sacs and pericardium. Through haematogenous spread, the organism reaches in the liver, spleen and kidneys where further replication occurs along with the production of reticulate and elementary bodies.

Characteristic symptoms

- Greenish diarrhoea
- Decrease in egg production
- Decreased fertility and hatchability

Macroscopic features

- Enlargement of spleen and liver with necrotic foci.
- Serofibrinous pericarditis.

- Air sacculitis, depositions of cheesy material.
- Greenish intestinal contents with catarrhal enteritis.

Microscopic features

- Necrosis and lymphoid aggregations in liver.
- Serofibrinous pericarditis.
- Catarrhal enteritis.

Diagnosis

- Symptoms and lesions
- Organism can be demonstrated in smears of spleen, liver, air sacs and stained with Giemsa stain
- Red coccoid elementary bodies
- Demonstration of chlamydial inclusions in liver cells in impression smear or tissue sections using special stain.

6

Pathology of Mycoplasmal Diseases

Chronic Respiratory Disease (CRD)

Chronic respiratory disease is caused by *Mycoplasma gallisepticum* and *E.coli* in birds under poor management and characterized by cloudy air sacs with thickening of their wall, accumulation of cheesy material in air sacs and lungs (Fig.6.1).

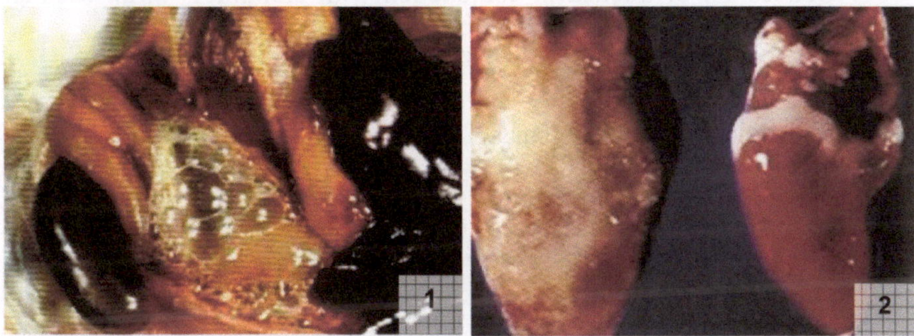

Fig. 6.1: Chronic respiratory disease caused by Mycoplasma gallisepticum and E.coli- (1) Cheesy material in air sacs and (2) Caseation in heart.

Etiology

- *Mycoplasma gallisepticum*
- *E.coli*
- Bad management like poor ventilation and inclement weather conditions
- Disease occurs more during winter and rainy season.

Pathogenesis

The disease is transmitted through direct contact of susceptible birds with infected carrier birds. It spreads through contaminated air, dust, droplets or feathers. It can also spread through infected eggs. The organism itself is not pathogenic but due to other pathogens like viruses of Ranikhet disease, Infectious bronchitis and Infectious bursal disease and the pathogenic strains of *E.coli* and *Haemophilus paragallinarum* may predispose the birds and make them susceptible for mycoplasma infection. Other factors include nutritional deficiency, excessive environmental dust and ammonia leads to the development of clinical signs and lesions.

Characteristic symptoms

- Gasping
- Gargling sound during respiration
- Frothy exudate in eyes with conjunctivitis

Macroscopic features

- Congestion of trachea in conjunction with cloudiness in air sacs and bronchial mucosa.
- Haemorrhage in trachea.
- Elongation of tracheal glands.

Diagnosis

- Symptoms and circumstantial evidences
- Lesions in air sacs and lungs.
- Immunological tests such as ELISA, tube agglutination plate agglutination test.
- Isolation of causative organisms
- Demonstration of organisms in tissue sections using special stains.

Infectious Synovitis

Infectious synovitis is a disease of adult birds caused by *Mycoplasma synoviae* and characterized by the presence of thick, creamy or cheesy material in synovial sac of hock joint, foot pad, keel bone and in air sacs (Fig.6.2).

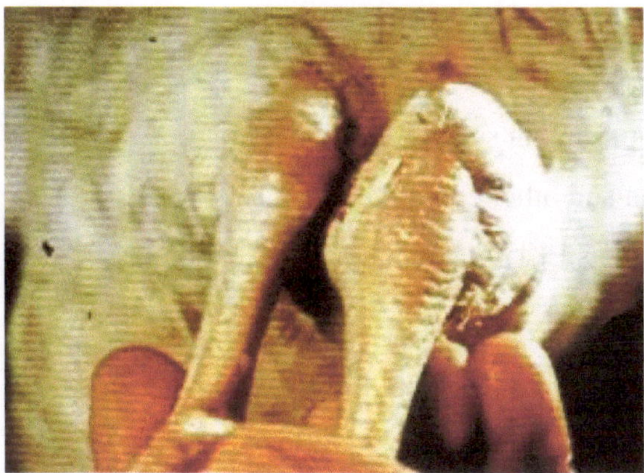

Fig. 6.2: Swelling of joints due to Mycoplasma synoviae.

Etiology

- *Mycoplasma synoviae*
- Some times complicated by *Pasteurella gallinarum*

Pathogenesis

It is transmitted through direct contact or through contaminated air, dust, droplets or feathers. After entry the organism causes mild respiratory disease and through haematogenous route, it reaches to different articular parts and respiratory tissues causing arthritis, respiratory distress, anemia and vasculitis.

Characteristic symptoms

- Swelling of foot pad and joints
- Pale comb
- Sulfur colour faeces

Macroscopic features

- Thick cheesy material in synovial sac of hock joints, foot pad, keel bone and air sacs.
- Greenish discoloration of liver.
- Hydropericardium

Microscopic features

- Lymphoid aggregation in synovial membrane, liver and air sacs.
- Catarrhal enteritis in duodenum.

Diagnosis

- Symptoms and lesions
- Demonstration of mycoplasma in synovial exudate.
- Isolation of mycoplasma and other causative organisms
- Immunological tests such as ELISA and plate agglutination test

7

Pathology of Spirochaetal Disease

Spirochetosis

Spirochetosis is caused by a spiral shaped organism *Borrelia anserina* and characterized by greenish diarrhoea, enlarged and mottled spleen, small necrotic patches on liver and linear haemorrhage in proventriculus. This disease is transmitted by a tick *Argas persicus* and thus also known as ***"tick fever"*** or ***"tick paralysis"***.

Etiology

- Spirochete *Borrelia anserina*
- Spiral shape 8-24m long and 0.2 to 0.3 m wide microorganism having 8-11 spirals.
- Stained with aniline dyes

Pathogenesis

Soft ticks of genus Argas are the main reservoir of the organism. *Borrelia anserina* can survive for long period either in birds or in environment. Birds become infected from saliva introduced by the tick on bite. After entry, the spirochaete reaches in blood circulation and cause septicemia with an abrupt and marked elevation of body temperature.

Characteristic symptoms

- Greenish diarrhoea
- Cyanosis of comb
- Jaundice

Macroscopic features

- Greenish diarrhoea with greenish intestinal contents.
- Cyanosis of comb.
- Enlargement of spleen with mottling.
- Enlargement of liver with small necrotic foci.
- Linear haemorrhage in proventriculus.
- Presence of ticks on skin / feather follicles.

Microscopic features

- Necrosis of hepatocytes.
- Necrosis and depletion of lymphoid tissue in spleen and haemosiderosis.
- Catarrhal enteritis.
- Perivascular gliosis in brain.
- Haemorrhagic dermatitis.
- Organism can be seen in liver sections by silver stain.

Diagnosis

- Symptoms and lesions
- Demonstration of spirochete in blood smears.
- Demonstration of ticks on skin during external examination.
- Demonstration of ticks in poultry house or on neighbouring plants.

8

Pathology of Fungal Diseases

Aspergillosis

Aspergillosis is a fungal disease of poultry caused by different species of *Aspergillus sp* and characterized by granulomatous nodules in lungs, thickening of air sacs and presence of fungal growth in lungs and air sacs in early age of chicks. It is also known as ***Brooders pneumonia*** (Fig.8.1).

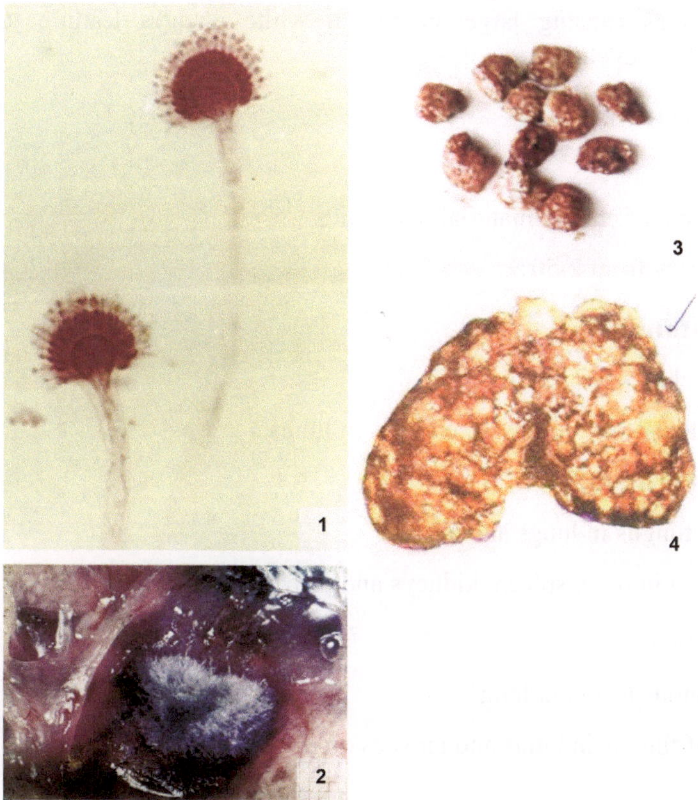

Fig. 8.1: Aspergillosis in poultry- **(1)** Aspergillus fumigatus, **(2)** Growth of fungus in air sacs and **(3&4)** Granulomatous lesions in lungs.

Etiology

- *Aspergillus fumigatus*
- *A. flavus*
- *A. nidulans*
- *A. glaucus*
- *A. niger*
- *A. candidus*

Pathogenesis

The disease is transmitted through inhalation of spores. The spores are deposited on conjunctiva, nasal and tracheal mucosa, lungs and air sacs and cause granuloma formation. Through hematogenous route it reaches in brain, pericardium, bone marrow, kidneys and other tissues. In brain, it produces lesions in meninges causing large superficial white plaques leading to ophthalmitis and iridocyclitis.

Characteristic symptoms

- Dyspnoea
- Accumulation of cheesy material in eye lids
- Mortality vary from 2-50%

Macroscopic features

- Lesions in chicks 5-7 days of age.
- Raised, pinhead size yellowish nodules in lungs.
- Thickening of air sacs.
- Growth of fungus in lungs and air sacs.
- Necrotic foci in liver, spleen, kidneys and proventriculus.

Microscopic features

- Granulomatous lesion in lungs.
- Presence of fungus in lungs and air sacs on microscopic examination.

Diagnosis

- Symptoms and lesions
- Demonstration of fungus in impression smear of lungs
- Cultures of fungus on SDA and its identification.
- Demonstration of fungus in lung tissue sections using special stains

Favus

Favus is a fungal disease of birds caused by *Trichophyton* sp. and characterized by deposition of thin, white flour like material on comb and skin of other featherless parts of body. It is also known as ***while comb disease***.

Etiology

- *Trichophyton magnini*

Pathogenesis

The disease is transmitted through contact or through contact with fomites. After superficial invasion of stratum corneum by hyphae, it causes epidermal hyperplasia and hyperkeratosis.

Characteristic symptoms

- Thin white flour like material deposits on comb
- Thickening of skin

Macroscopic features

- White, flour like material deposits on comb and skin
- Necrotic foci on trachea and oesophagus.
- Scab formation on skin.

Microscopic features

- Fungus in skin scab and scrapings of skin
- Granulomatous lesions in skin.

Diagnosis

- Symptoms and lesions
- Presence of fungus and its identification.
- Isolation and identification of fungus

Candidiasis

Candidiasis is a fungal disease of poultry which occurs sporadically and caused by *Candida* sp. and characterized by Turkish towel like appearance of crop, oesophagus and ulcers in mouth and oesophagus. It is also known as ***thrush***.

Etiology

- *Candida albicans*
- *Monilia albicans*

Pathogenesis

The fungus is acquired by ingestion of contaminated materials. Then the fungus becomes part of normal flora of mouth, oesophagus and crop. When there is immunosuppression, the fungus proliferates and penetrates epithelial surface leading to the stimulation of the epithelial hyperplasia and diphtheritic membrane formation.

Characteristic symptoms

- Stunted growth of birds
- Ruffled feathers

Macroscopic features

- Turkish towel like lesions in crop and/or oesophagus.
- Congestion in proventriculus.
- Ulcers in mouth and oesophagus.

Microscopic features

- Granulomatous lesions in crop and oesophagus.
- Fungal colony in tissues.

Diagnosis

- Symptoms and lesions
- Fungus in impression smears of affected organ / tissue.
- Isolation and identification of fungus.

Histoplasmosis

Histoplasmosis is a sporadic fungal disease of birds caused by *Histoplasma* sp. and characterized by granulomatous lesions in liver and other parts of body.

Etiology

- *Histoplasma capsulatum*

Pathogenesis

Infection spreads through inhalation of spores present in soil or dusty environment of the poultry house. The fungus settles in lungs and proliferates within the macrophages and spreads in other visceral organs.

Characteristic symptoms

- Diarrhoea
- Soiling of cloaca with semisolid cheesy material

Macroscopic features

- Presence of round, raised, rough granulomatous lesions on liver, spleen and other organs.

Microscopic features

- Granulomatous lesions in liver.
- Presence of round or oval yeast like fungal spores in tissues.

Diagnosis

- Symptoms and lesions
- Isolation and identification of fungus.
- Demonstration of fungus in affected tissue using special stains

Aflatoxicosis

Aflatoxicosis is a toxic condition of poultry widely prevalent in all parts of the country caused by fungal toxins and characterized by hepatic lesions, immunosuppression and cancer (Fig.8.2).

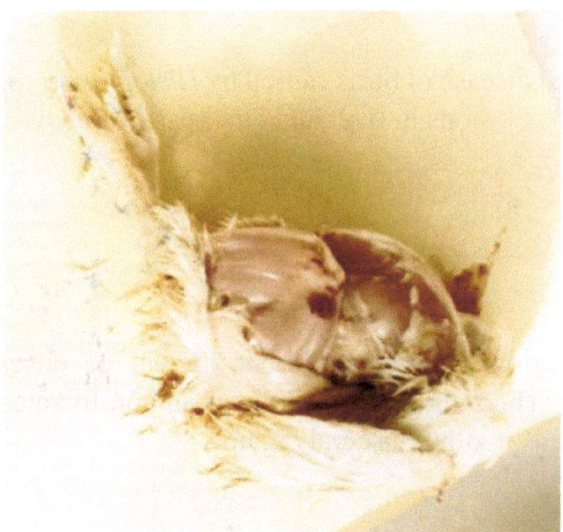

Fig. 8.2: Haemorrhage in muscle of bird due to Aflatoxicosis.

Etiology

- Fungal toxins of *Aspergillus flavus* and *Penicillium puberlum* and several other fungi.
- Aflatoxin B_1, B_2, G_1, G_2.

Pathogenesis

After ingestion aflatoxin, under goes biotransformation into highly reactive metabolites which binds with nucleic acids and reduce protein synthesis and causes immunosuppression. These metabolic alterations cause enlargement of liver, spleen and kidneys and atrophy of bursa of Fabricious, thymus and testicular tissues.

Characteristic symptoms

- Enlargement of abdomen
- Anemia
- Drop in egg production
- Spasms of neck muscles and arched back
- Retarded growth of birds

Macroscopic features

- Enlargement of liver
- Necrotic foci in liver.

- Congestion and haemorrhage in liver.
- Tumourous nodules in liver.
- Atrophy of spleen.
- Haemorrhage in muscles.
- Loose attachment of mucosa of Gizzard.
- Loss of production of eggs.

Microscopic features

- Necrosis in hepatic parenchyma.
- Proliferation of bile duct epithelium.
- Fibrosis in liver.
- Haemorrhage in muscles and myocardium.

Diagnosis

- Symptoms and lesions
- Detection of toxins in poultry feed/tissues of affected birds using TLC or flurotoxinometer.
- Immunodiagnostic tests for detection of aflatoxins in feed and tissues.
- ELISA
- DIA

Ochratoxicosis

Ochratoxicosis is a toxic condition of poultry caused by a fungal toxin and characterized by nephrosis, visceral gout, pale bone marrow and haemorrhage in intestines.

Etiology

- Ochratoxins produced by *Aspergillus ochraceous* and several other species of *Aspergillus* and *Penicillium* sp.

Pathogenesis

Ochratoxin is found in maize and in most of the small grains contaminated with moulds. It inhibits protein synthesis, produces acute proximal tubular epithelial necrosis in kidneys and inhibits normal renal uric acid excretion.

Characteristic symptoms

- Anemia
- Increased clotting time
- Loss of pigmentation

Macroscopic features

- Enlargement of kidneys
- Deposition of urates on kidneys
- Hemorrhage in kidneys
- Ureters distended due to accumulation of urates.
- Hemorrhage in duodenum.
- Anemia
- Pale bone marrow.
- Atrophy of lymphoid organs
- Ascites

Microscopic features

- Nephrosis, deposition of urates.
- Infiltration of heterophils and fibrosis.
- Hemorrhage in intestinal wall.
- Lymphoid depletion in bursa, thymus and spleen.

Diagnosis

- Symptoms and lesions
- Detection of ochratoxin in poultry feed/tissues using TLC/HPLC methods.
- Immunodiagnostic tests for detection of toxins in feed
- ELISA
- DIA

Trichothecene toxicity

Trichothecene toxicosis occurs in poultry as a result of feeding of contaminated feed caused by mycotoxin trichothecene and characterized by gastroenteritis, immunosuppression and death.

Etiology

- Mycotoxins – Trichothecene having following components:
  - Deoxynivalenol (DON) or Vomitoxin
  - T- 2 toxin
  - Diacetoxyscirpenol (DAS).
  - Satratoxin, roridin, verrucarin.
- Of these, DON is most common contaminant of corn, wheat and other grains.
- T -2 toxin and DAS are sporadic.
- Produced by fungus-*Fusarium* spp, *Trichothecium* spp, *Myrothecium* Spp, and *Cephalosporium* Spp.

Pathogenesis

- Enters in body through ingestion.
- Absorbed through intestine, causing damage to intestinal epithelial cells.
- Inhibits protein synthesis.
- Leads to gastroenteritis, immunosuppression.

Clinical Manifestation

- Diarrhoea, Melena
- Stomatitis.
- Hyperkeratosis.
- Ulceration on skin.

Macroscopic feathers

- Stomatitis, ulcers in oesophagus.
- Necrosis of G.I. tract mucosa.

- Ulcers on Skin.
- Hyperkeratosis.

Microscopic features

- Gastroenteritis, necrosis of epithelium of intestines.
- Hyperkeratosis
- Lymphoid depletion in spleen.
- Lymphopenia, Pancytopenia.

Diagnosis

- Symptoms and lesions.
- Detection of toxins in feed, tissue, blood.

9

Pathology of Parasitic Diseases

Roundworms (Nematodes)

1. *Ascaridia galli*

A. galli is the common roundworm of poultry seen in intestines at the time of necropsy. This parasite may cause retardation of growth, loss of egg production, catarrhal enteritis and sometimes mortality due to obstruction of gut (Fig.9.1).

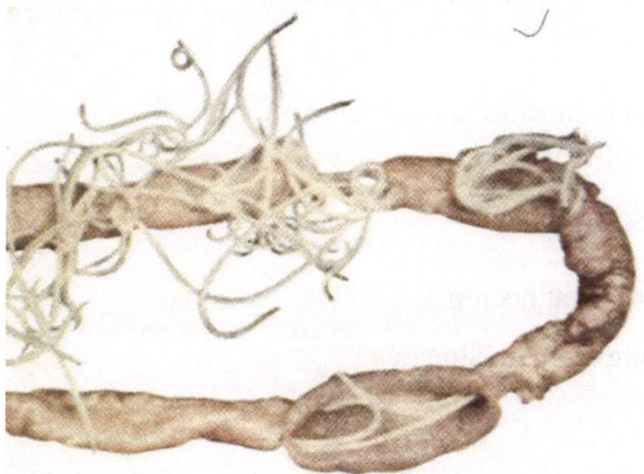

Fig. 9.1: Ascaridia galli in intestine.

Etiology

- *A. galli* parasites are grey, thread like 5-10 cm in length.
- Eggs are elliptical with thick and shiny wall.

Pathogenesis

Transmission occurs through faecal - oral route. The eggs may survive for several months in litter and they take at least 10-15 days to develop the infective stage. The eggs of parasites hatch in proventriculus or intestine to develop fully grown parasite within 40-50 days.

Characteristic symptoms

- Growth retardation
- Anemia
- Decreased egg production

Macroscopic features

- Anemia
- Emaciation
- Presence of *A. galli* in intestines
- Catarrhal enteritis

Microscopic features

- Presence of parasitic section in the lumen of intestine
- Catarrhal enteritis
- Eosinophilic infiltration in mucosa and sub mucosa

Diagnosis

- Symptoms and lesions
- Presence of parasites in gut at necropsy
- Examination of droppings for parasitic ova.

2. *Syngamus trachea*

- Affects growers
- Causes emaciation
- 'Y' shape red worms present in trachea

3. *Gongylonema ingluvicola*

- Worms in crop under mucosa
- Causes emaciation and retardation of growth

4. *Dispharynx nasuta* and *Tetrameres pattersoni*

- Diarrhoea, emaciation
- Hemorrhage in proventriculus
- Worms in proventricular glands

5. *Cheilospirura hamulosa*

- Emaciation
- Necrotic nodules in gizzard, presence of worms
- Hemorrhage in gizzard

6. *Heterakis gallinarum (Fig.9.2)*

- Emaciation
- Typhlitis
- Presence of worms in caeca

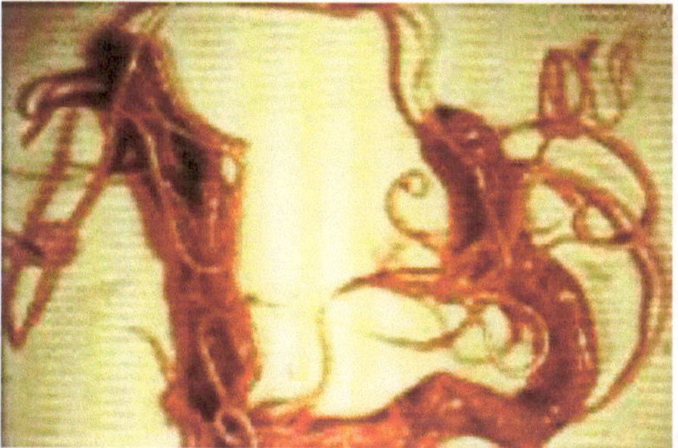

Fig. 9.2: Heterakis gallinarum in caecum.

7. *Capillaria annulata (Fig.9.3)*

- Filamentous worm of poultry
- Esophagitis

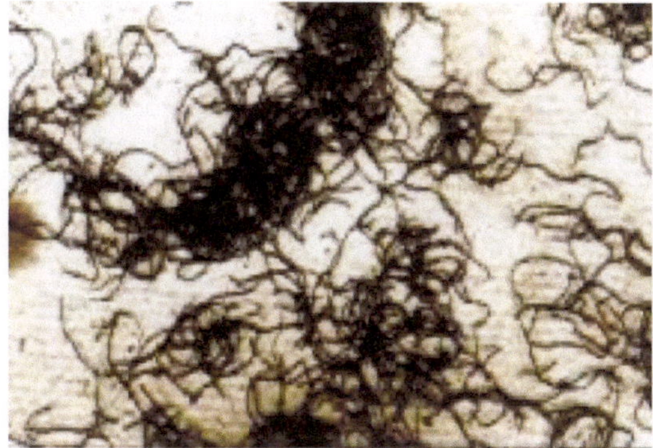

Fig. 9.3: *Capillaria* sp. worms in intestine.

Tape worms (Cestodes)

Avian cestodes are thin, white tape worms present in gut causing enteritis and melena leading to retardation of growth (Fig.9.4).

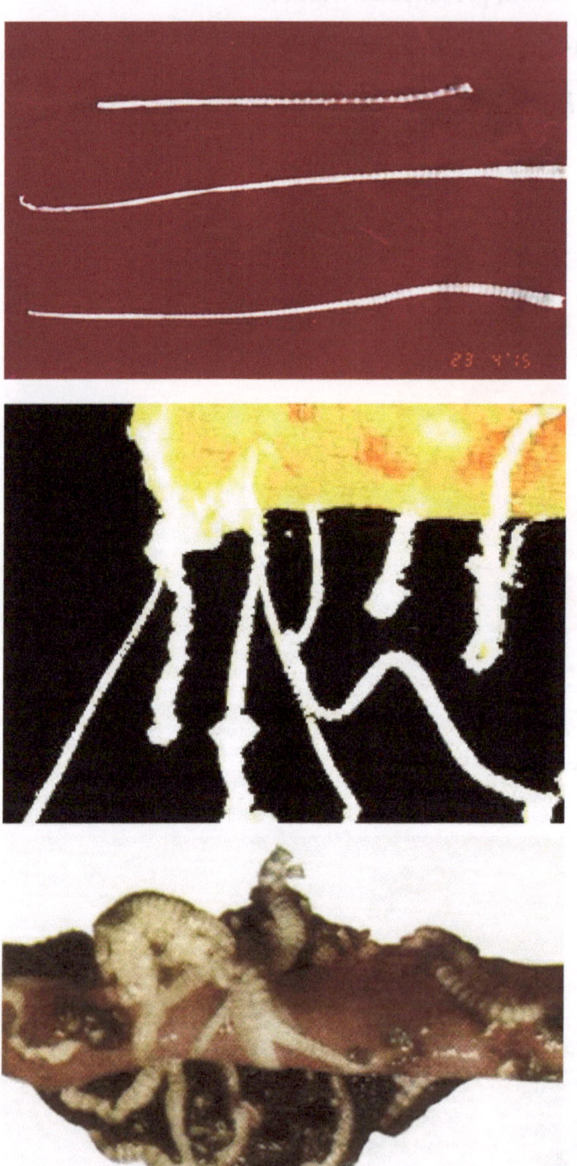

Fig. 9.4: Tape worm infection in poultry- **(1)** Raillietina tetragona and **(2&3)** Tapeworms in intestine

Etiology

- *Davainea proglottina* (3 mm in length)
- *Choanotaenia infundibulum, Raillietina tetragona* and *R. echinobothrida* (25-30 cm in length)

Pathogenesis

Transmission occurs through slugs, flies and ants infected with segments of parasites. It penetrates mucosa of intestine to cause hemorrhagic enteritis and forms nodules visible from outside of the intestines.

Characteristic symptoms

- Emaciation
- Weakness
- Red droppings due to mixing of blood

Macroscopic features

- Catarrhal and hemorrhagic enteritis
- Granulomatous nodules in wall of intestine

Microscopic features

- Catarrhal and hemorrhagic enteritis

Diagnosis

- Symptoms and lesions
- Presence of parasite in gut at necropsy
- Presence of parasitic segments in droppings

Flat worms (Trematodes)

Trematodes are flat worms rarely found in birds. Some of the important flat worms are:

1. *Prosthogonymus macrorchis*
2. *Echinostoma revolutum*
3. *Echinoparyphium recurvatum*
4. *Prosthogonymus indicus*
5. *Catatropis indica*

Ectoparasites

Common ectoparasites including ticks, mites and lice of poultry are:

1. Ticks

a. *Argas persicus*

b. *Aegyptianella pullorum*

2. Mites

a. *Dermanyssus gallinae*- Red mite

b. *Syringophilus bipectinatus*- Feather mite

c. *Knemidocotes gallinae*- Feather mite

d. *K. mutans*- Scaly leg mite

e. *Cytodites nudus*- Air sac mite

Protozoan parasites

1. Coccidiosis

Coccidiosis is caused by protozoan parasites of *Eiemeria* sp. and characterized by hemorrhagic enteritis and mortality in chickens (Fig.9.5).

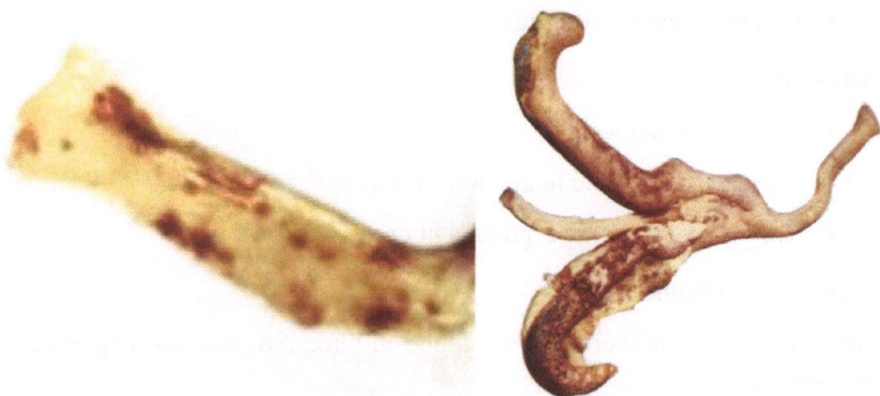

Fig. 9.5: Coccidiosis in poultry-**(1)** Intestinal and **(2)** Caecal coccidiosis.

Etiology

- Intestinal form
- *Eimeria acervulina*

- *E. necatrix*
- *E. maxima*
- *E. brunetti*
- *E. preacox*
- *E. mitis*
- *E. hagani*
- *E. mivati*
- Caecal coccidiosis
- *E. tenella*

Pathogenesis

Oocysts with sporozoites are ingested by birds through contaminated feed, water or litter. The sporozoites are released and penetrate epithelial cells of villi and develop into round bodies (trophozoites). It then grows to form first generation schizont, nuclei of which have sickle shape and known as merozoites. The merozoites after breaking schizonts can start second cycle to form second generation schizonts. After 2-3 cycle, the merozoites develop sexual phage to form male (micro gametocytes) and female (macro gametocytes) cells. The micro gametes penetrate and fuse with macro gametes resulting in fertilization and formation of oocysts which are liberated in intestinal lumen and pass out along with faeces. A single ingested oocyst can develop into millions of oocysts in a bird.

Characteristic symptoms

- Emaciation and anemia
- Retarded growth
- Blood mixed droppings
- Mortality upto 50%

Macroscopic features

- Hemorrhagic enteritis
- Typhlitis
- Thickening of intestinal wall

Microscopic features

- Catarrhal and hemorrhagic enteritis
- Presence of coccidia in intestinal sections

Diagnosis

- Symptoms and lesions
- Examination of droppings or intestinal scrapings for the presence of coccidia.

Histomoniasis

Histomoniasis is a disease of growers caused by protozoan parasite *Histomonas* sp. and characterized by necrotic ulcers in caeca and necrotic foci in liver. It is also known as ***black head*** disease (Fig.9.6).

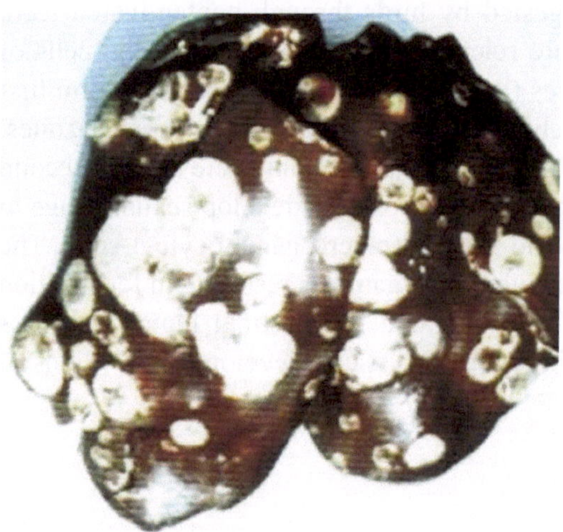

Fig. 9.6: Histomonas meleagredis infection in poultry- necrotic lesions in liver.

Etiology

- *Histomonas meleagredis*
- Round, vacuolated cytoplasm with single nucleus.

Pathogenesis

Transmission of protozoan parasite occurs through faecal contamination of feed and water or through earthworm, flies and eggs of *Heterakis gallinarum*. Parasite enters in wall of caeca and causes lesions.

Characteristic symptoms

- Diarrhoea with sulfur colour faeces
- Icterus

Macroscopic features

- Necrotic ulcers in caeca
- Circular, concave, green necrotic foci (1 cm diameter) in liver

Microscopic features

- Necrosis in liver
- Presence of protozoan parasite (unicellular 8-13 µl, with four flagella)

Diagnosis

- Symptoms and lesions
- Microscopic examination of caecal contents/scrapings.

Trichomoniasis

Trichomoniasis is a protozoan parasitic disease characterized by formation of yellow round nodules in esophagus and crop of pigeons (Fig.9.7).

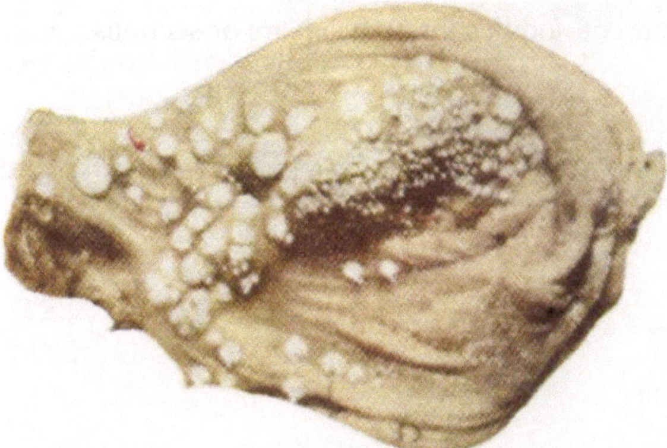

Fig. 9.7: Trichomoniasis in crop of poultry.

Etiology

- *Trichomonas gallinae*

Pathogenesis

Organism is transmitted directly from infected birds to newly hatched pigeons. Small yellowish necrotic lesions develop in oral cavity specially on soft palate after 3-14 days of infection which further spreads to oesophagus, crop, proventriculus, liver, lungs and intestines.

Characteristic symptoms

- Emaciation
- Accumulation of greenish fluid or cheesy material in mouth and crop
- Pendulous crop

Macroscopic features

- Yellow, button shaped necrotic foci in mouth, oesophagus and crop

Microscopic features

- Necrosis
- Presence of protozoan parasites in sections of oesophagus and crop

Diagnosis

- Symptoms and lesions
- Microscopic examination of nodules through smears or sections.

Hexamitiasis

Hexamitiasis is a protozoan parasitic disease of turkey poults of about 4-6 weeks characterized by diarrhoea and mortality.

Etiology

- *Hexamita meleagridis*
- Almond shaped parasite

Pathogenesis

The source of infection is adult carrier birds. On ingestion it produces catarrhal enteritis with bulbous areas containing watery contents on duodenum and jejunum.

Characteristic symptoms

- Diarrhoea
- Loss of weight and death

Macroscopic features

- Bulbous nodules in intestine

Microscopic features

- Presence of protozoan parasites in caecum, duodenum and bursa

Diagnosis

- Symptoms and lesions
- Microscopic examination of lesion/caeca for parasites

10

Pathology of Vices and Miscellaneous Disease Conditions

Cannibalism

Cannibalism is a bad habit of birds in which the birds attack their fellow birds and eat their flesh. It is done through sharp end of beak, which causes deep wounds specially on vent. Sometimes the wounds are so deep that leads to death of affected bird. Two types of cannibalism vices are common i.e. vent pecking and feather pecking.

Cause / Predisposing Factors

- Over crowding
- Genetic predisposition
- Hemorrhage in external genitalia
- Protein deficiency (arginine and methionine deficiency)
- Loss of feathers
- Wounds
- Prolapse of cloaca

Egg Eating

Sometimes a bird develops habit of eating its own eggs. This problem may start with the presence of broken eggs in poultry house and birds develop a taste for it.

Pica

Birds eat non food items such as feathers, litter material, threads, mud, bangle (Fig. 10.1) etc. It may occur due to phosphorus deficiency, parasitic load in gut, new litter material or poor managemental conditions.

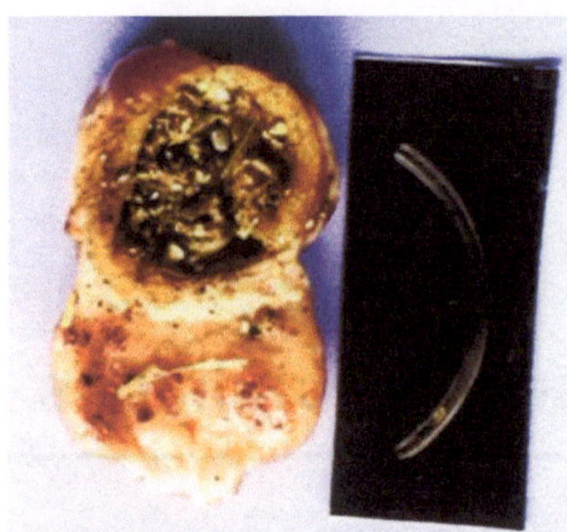

Fig. 10.1: Pica in poultry- Presence of a piece of bangle in proventriculus and gizzard.

Heat Stroke

The presence of thick layers of feathers on body of bird and absence of sweat glands on skin makes the birds more susceptible to heat stroke in summer season. Inadequate water supply, absence of trees/vegetation around poultry houses, overcrowding, poor ventilation, etc. may predispose the birds for heat stroke which is characterized by open beak; panting (Fig. 10.2), paralysis, congestion and hemorrhage in brain along with dehydration.

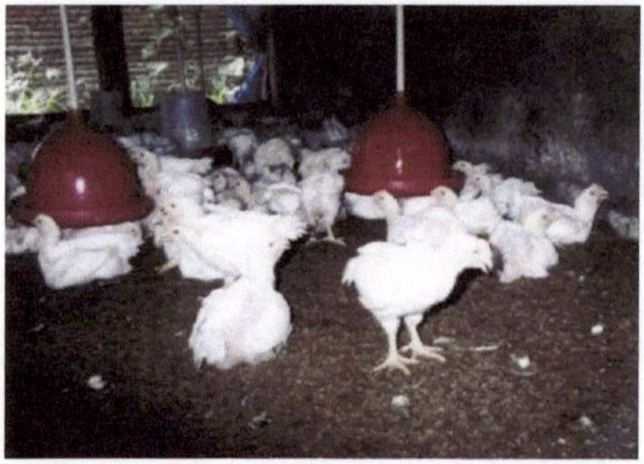

Fig. 10.2: Panting in poultry due to heat stroke.

Prolapse of Cloaca

The prolapse of cloaca has been observed due to fusariotoxins which increases the peristalsis in layers. It may enhance the cannibalism in birds.

Impaction of Crop

Sometimes birds may eat litter material (Fig. 10.3), grass, feathers, fibrous food, nails, pieces of sticks, stumps of feathers which causes impaction in crop. If the nail having sharp edge, it may penetrate and cause ingluvitis and/ or proventriculitis (Fig. 10.4).

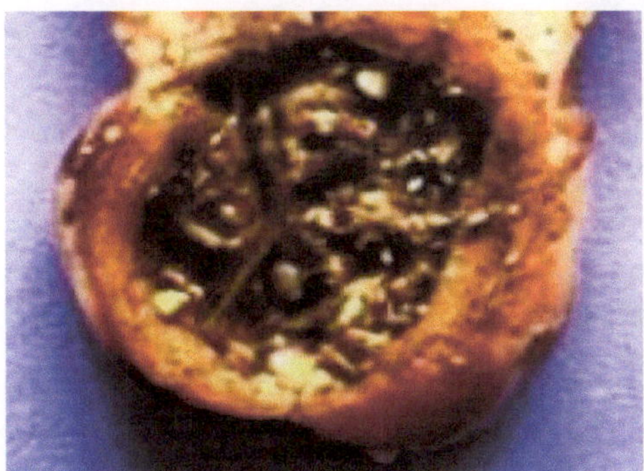

Fig. 10.3: Impaction of crop due to litter material.

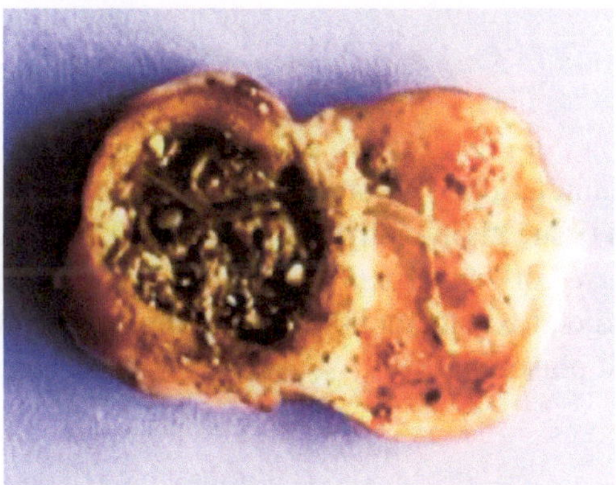

Fig. 10.4: Proventriculitis due to bangle.

Egg Bound Condition

Egg bound condition is inability of a layer bird to expel a normal egg. It may occur in new laying hens due to paralysis of nerves of oviduct or its inflammation that leads to prolapse. The egg remains in oviduct and death occurs in such birds. Sometimes, eggs from ovary do not reach in oviduct and drops in peritoneal cavity leading to egg borne peritonitis (Fig. 10.5).

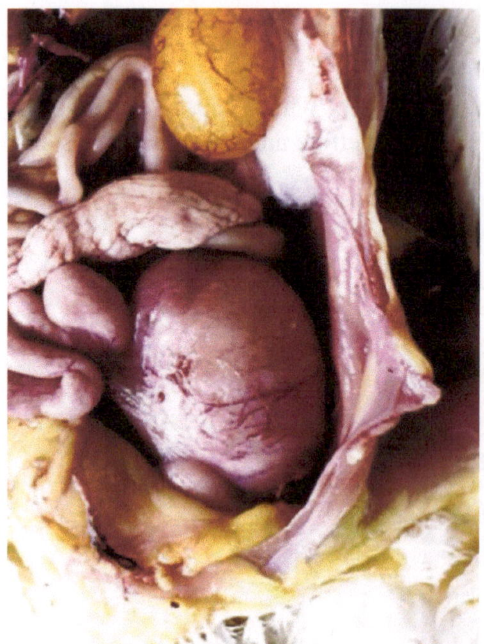

Fig. 10.5: Egg borne peritonitis in a bird.

Toxic Fat Syndrome

In this condition, birds show accumulation of water in abdominal cavity, pericardial sac and in subcutaneous tissue giving jelly like appearance. This is also known as "***chick oedema disease***" or "***water belly***". It may be associated with phosphorus deficient soybean diet, toxic factor associated with fat in feed and carbon monoxide, dioxin or salt poisoning.

Gout

Gout is deposition of uric acid and urates in kidneys, heart, ureters and other internal organs. It may occur due to excess of protein, deficiency of vitamin A, infectious bursal disease, infectious bronchitis, aflatoxicosis, orchratoxicosis and other diseases involving kidneys. In this conditions, one may find chalky/ sandy material on touch on the surface of the organs (Fig. 10.6).

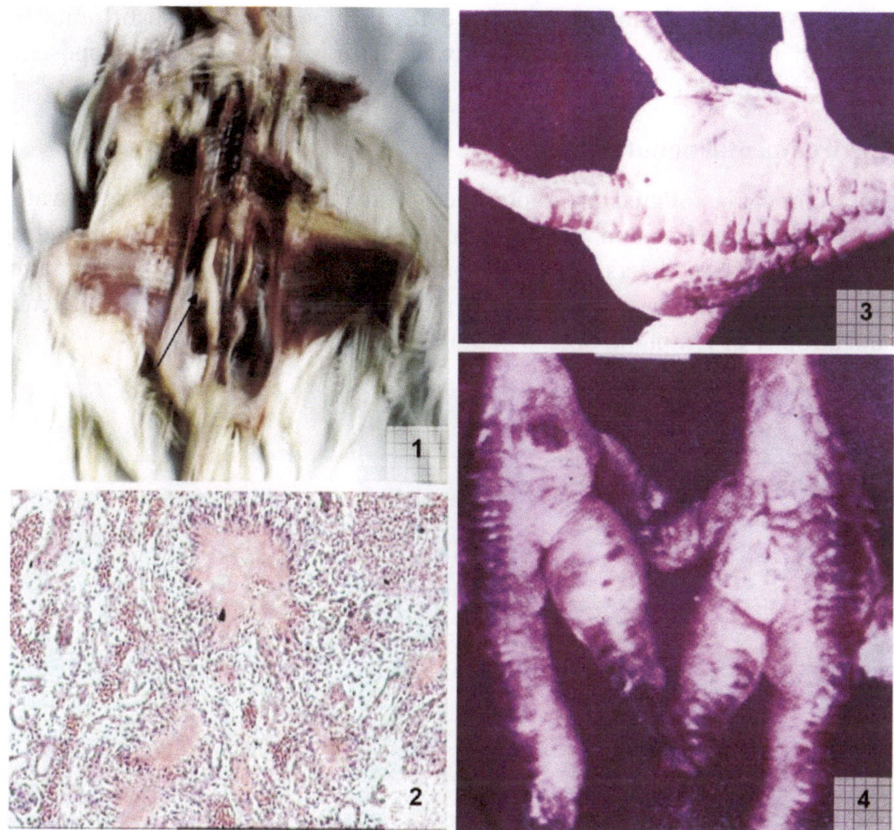

Fig. 10.6: Gout in poultry- **(1)** Deposition of urates on heart and kidneys, **(2)** Histological features of gout, and **(3&4)** Swelling of paw and claws.

Fatty Liver and Kidney Syndrome

Fatty liver and kidney syndrome (FLKS) is characterized by pale or yellowish liver with petechiae, pale heart and kidneys and hydropericardium. It may occur due to biotin deficiency, inadequate feeding, protein deficiency and stress as a result of noise, excessive cold or heat, power failure etc.

Fatty Liver Syndrome

It is characterized by enlarged, yellowish, friable liver with rupture and internal haemorrhage. This condition is associated with faulty diet or stress of high egg production.This is also known as fatty liver hemorrhagic syndrome.

Blue comb Disease

This is also known as avian monocytosis and is characterized by bluish colour of comb, increased number of monocytes in blood, deposition of urates in kidneys, and atrophy of spleen. The exact cause is not known but supposedly occurs due to some nutritional factors or viral etiology.

Environmental pollutants

Environment is polluted due to presence of unwanted materials in food, water, air and surroundings of poultry, particularly by agrochemicals including pesticides and fertilizers5 The environmental pollutants exert their direct or indirect effect on the poultry health and production leading to immunodeficiency and atrophy of lymphoid organs in poultry (Fig.10.7).

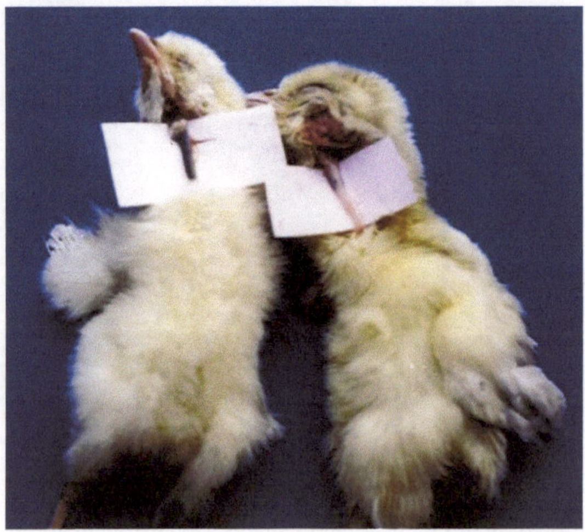

Fig. 10.7: Deposition of generator emitted smoke carbon in trachea of chicks.

Vent gleet

Vent gleet is caused by *Candida albicans* and Characterized by the presence of whitish discharge fermenting like yeast at Vent, missing feathers, congested and oedematous skin and crusting on feathers. It may lead to depression, loss of egg production, loss of weight and diarrhea.

Internal layer

Internal layer means the presence of partially or fully formed eggs in abdominal cavity due to reverse peristalsis of the oviduct. Such eggs are often misshapen and with partial or complete absorption of contents and absence of shell. This condition is also kanoon as defective egg syndrome. Such birds also contribute to non-performance / production losses of the farm.

Breast Blister

It is sternal bursitis; when bursa becomes inflamed due to trauma or infection, fluid accumulates and appears as a fluid filled blister of 1-3 cm diameter size. It occurs due to poor feathering, hard flooring and leg weakness. Infectious agents involved may be *Staphylococcus*, *Pasteurella*, *Mycoplasma* etc.

Ascites Syndrome

Ascites is the accumulation of fluid in peritoneal cavity, it is often transudate. It may occur due to increased vascular hydraulic pressure and is associated with hepatic fibrosis, pulmonary hypertension, aflatoxins, *Clostridium perfringens*, Salt poisoning etc.

Cage layer fatigue

Cage layer fatigue is like osteoporosis, occurs in caged chickens as a result of high egg production. Lack of exercise is also a cause of this condition. It may occur in birds due to calcium deficient diet. In older birds, it is associated with deficiency of phosphorus and /or vitamin D3. In this condition birds are unable to stand on their feet and are having fragile bones. Affected birds lie down and not eating feed. Egg shells become thin.

Round heart disease

Round heart disease is having unknown etiology but possibly due to Salmonellosis and characterised by myodegeneration, deformity of heart and sudden death. It is accompanied by ascites, hydropericardium and congestion of visceral organs. It is also Known as cardiomyopathy.

Impaction of oviduct

Oviduct is impacted due to infection, oedema, inflammation and /or large size ova. It may result loss of production. Eggs get accumulated in the oviduct, which swells and puts endue pressure leading to break/burst. It may further result in cystic hyperplasia of oviduct. Eggs are sometimes produced too big such as double yolked eggs. It may be due to infectious bronchitis virus, and / or *E coli* infection.

False layer

False layer poultry ovulate normally but their yolk is dropped in abdominal cavity rather than being collected in oviduct. It may be due to inflammation, oedema and obstruction of the oviduct caused by *E.coli* and/or *Mycoplasma* Spp. The yolk is absorbed from the abdominal cavity and birds remain normal without showing any clinical symptoms except not laying eggs, Hyperplasia of ovary and oviduct due to infectious bronchitis virus. Atrophy of ovary due to stress or mycotoxins may be the other cause of false layer.

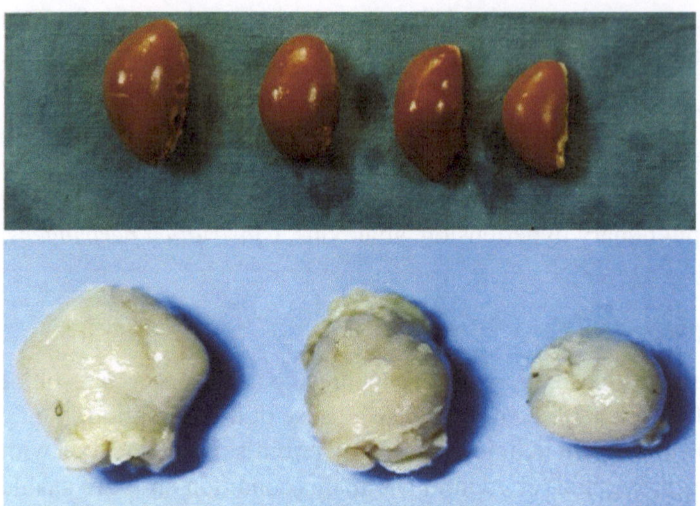

Fig. 10.8: Atrophy of lymphoid organs due to pesticides and heavy metals in feed and water.

Index